antony worrall thompson's

GLdiet
made simple

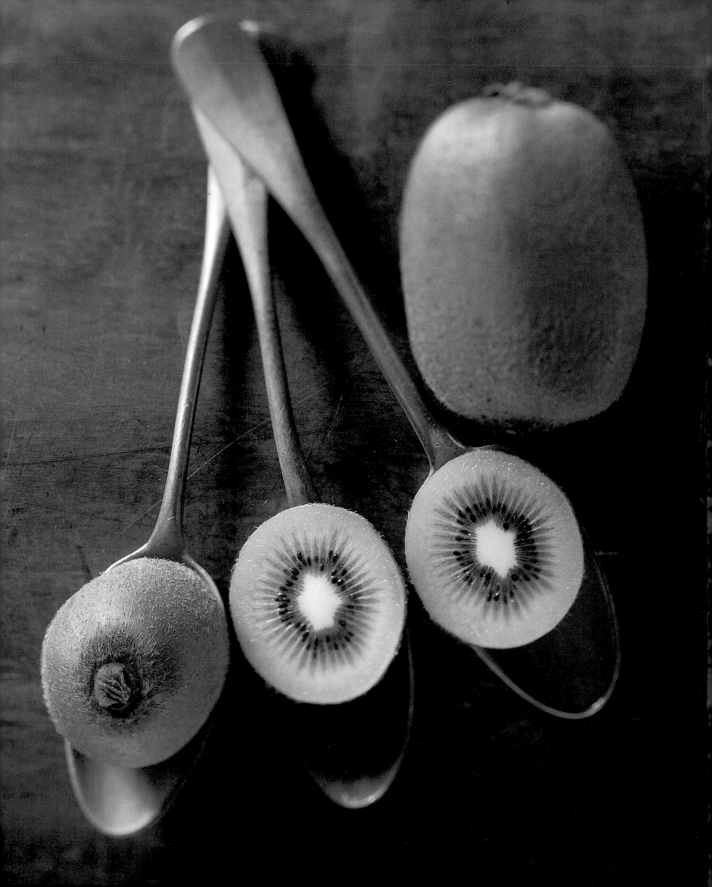

antony worrall thompson's
GLdiet
made simple

with Dr Mabel Blades & Jane Suthering

Photography by Steve Lee

KYLE CATHIE LTD

To Trevor, our gorgeous golden retriever, whom we sadly lost recently.

First published in Great Britain in 2006 by
Kyle Cathie Limited
122 Arlington Road
London NW1 7HP
general.enquiries@kyle-cathie.com
www.kylecathie.com

10 9 8 7 6 5 4 3 2 1

ISBN-13: 978 1 85626 662 8
ISBN-10: 1 85626 662 1

Editorial Director Muna Reyal
Designer Alison Fenton
Photographer Steve Lee assisted by Tony Briscoe
Home Economist Jane Suthering assisted by Anna Helm
Styling Jo Harris
Copyeditor Hilary Mandleberg
Editorial Assistant Cecilia Desmond
Recipe Analysis Dr Mabel Blades
Production Sha Huxtable and Alice Holloway

A Cataloguing In Publication record for this title is available from the British Library.

Colour reproduction by Sang Choy
Printed and bound in Singapore by KHL Printing Co.

Important note
The information and advice contained in this book are intended as a general guide to dieting and healthy eating and are not specific to individuals or their particular circumstances. This book is not intended to replace treatment by a qualified practitioner. Neither the authors nor the publishers can be held responsible for claims arising from the inappropriate use of any dietary regime.

Do not attempt self-diagnosis or self-treatment for serious or long-term conditions without consulting a medical professional or qualified practitioner.

Acknowledgments
There are too many people to thank but certain individuals deserve a special mention:

To my brilliant, good-humoured wife, Jacinta and our two children, Toby and Billie, who acted unknowingly as guinea pigs for many of the recipes. To Blake and Sam, my strapping Aussie sons, whose bodies I aspire to!

To Dr Mabel Blades and Jane Suthering for their excellent involvement in this book. They have worked very hard.

To Kyle and her superb team at Kyle Cathie, including Muna Reyal, my editor, for giving me the opportunity to produce this cookbook. Also thanks to Alison Fenton, the designer, who did an excellent job. They turned my offerings into a beautifully executed book.

To Louise Townsend, my energetic and ultra-efficient PA, who fielded hundreds of telephone calls from the publishers and who was regularly on hand to smooth troubled waters when the pressures of deadlines occasionally took their toll.

To Fiona Lindsay, Linda Shanks and Lesley Turnbull at Limelight Management who are constantly there to make sure I have more than enough work to handle.

To David Wilby, my business partner, and my head chefs and managers at all my restaurants who kept the boat afloat in my often-extended absences, Issa, George, Candido and Antonio, Richard, Alethia and Will.

And finally, Steve Lee also deserves a special mention for his terrific photos that really do the recipes justice.

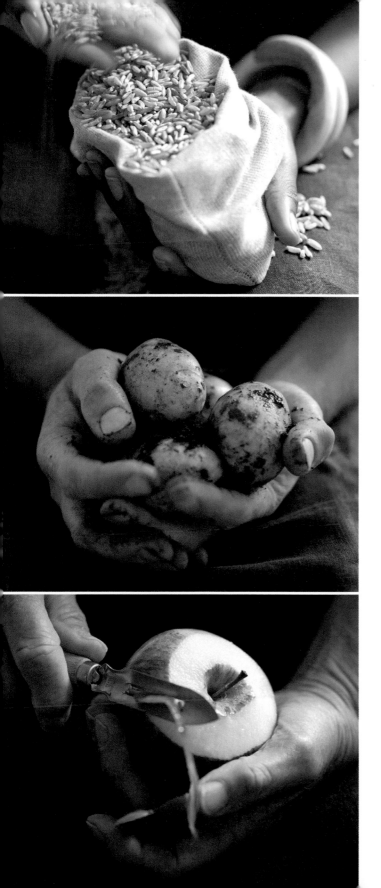

Contents

Introduction 6
How to lose weight permanently 8
The role of carbohydrates 10
The Glycaemic Load 12
Calculating the GL 13
Losing weight 14
The GL and weight loss 15
Zero-rated GL foods 16
The benefits of the GL diet 18
How the GL diet can help with
    health problems 19
Reducing the GL of a meal 20
The GL diet and shopping 21
The GI and GL food table 22
About the recipes 26
Low GL meal ideas 28
GL meal plans 30

THE RECIPES

Grains and flours 33
Pulses 49
Nuts and seeds 63
Vegetables 75
Eggs and dairy 89
Meat and poultry 99
Fish and shellfish 115
Fruit 129
Sweet treats 141

Index 156
Conversion table 158
Acknowledgements & Resources 159

Introduction

When I was diagnosed with Syndrome X or metabolic syndrome, a pre-diabetic state, a few years ago, I made it my mission to prove that you could still eat good, healthy food without it being boring, food that even those who were not diabetic could actually enjoy.

It all started with *Healthy Eating For Diabetes* which was such a success that I researched the GI (glycaemic index) diet further. Last year saw the publication of *Antony Worrall Thompson's GI Diet* and little did I know when I started to write it that it would be the diet of 2005.

But the GI diet should be seen as diet with a small 'd' as it's more of a lifestyle change; it is something we should all be doing, whether we have diabetes or not. All too often, our modern way of eating is based on sugar-based simple carbohydrates which are rapidly absorbed, raising your blood sugar levels rapidly only for them to go into free-fall a couple of hours later, causing hunger pangs as well as an extremely detrimental effect on our health. What we all need to eat are foods with a low GI and GL that the body absorbs slowly, making us feel full for much longer and keeping our blood sugar levels constant.

The GL (Glycaemic Load) Diet Made Simple is the third book in my series, based on the GI diet. It takes the diet one step further by balancing foods on the plate, looking at portion sizes which the GI doesn't do. For instance, carrots have a medium GI but its rating is based on 500g which of course you wouldn't eat in one portion. The GL calculates the glucose effect of a normal portion size, say 80g, which means that the glycaemic load is in fact very low.

The real success of this diet is not just about losing weight but more important keeping it off. Working with Mabel Blades and Jane Suthering, I have looked at other healthy aspects of eating, sodium and fat levels as well as calories, of course. We've packed the book full of necessary facts as well as over 100 great recipes and you don't have to do the calculation from GI to GL as it is too complicated for everyday use; we like to keep it simple so we've made all the necessary calculations for you. Read the facts then enjoy the recipes and live a healthy life.

OPPOSITE, TOP ROW, LEFT TO RIGHT: whole grain flour, new potatoes and sweet potato, wild rice, camargue red rice, brown basmati rice. MIDDLE ROW, LEFT TO RIGHT: bananas, curd cheese, coconut. BOTTOM ROW, LEFT TO RIGHT: walnuts, aubergine, buckwheat, quinoa and bulgur.

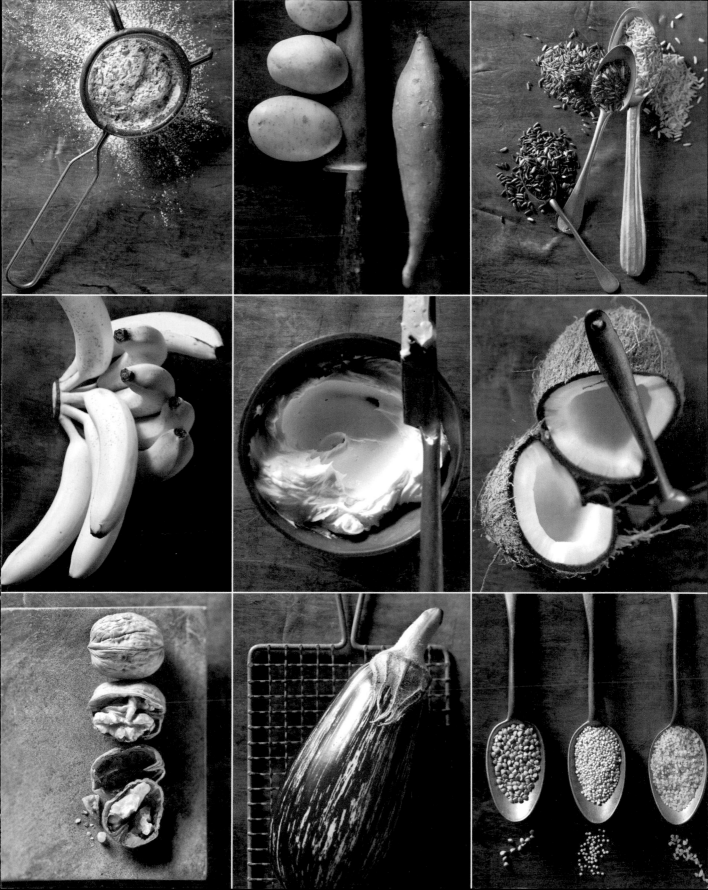

How to lose weight permanently

The problems of being overweight have been well publicised recently. We are also starting to understand that unhealthy diets can lead to obesity, digestive problems such as irritable bowel syndrome, some cancers and coronary heart disease. Many of us try to lose weight and succeed, but then find that the lost pounds just seem to come straight back again, plus a bit more. When that happens, it's often difficult to have another go at losing the weight. What anyone wanting to lose weight needs is a new way of eating for life rather than a short-term fix, and that new way of eating must be healthy, full of variety and leave them feeling satisfied.

A healthy diet – whether you're losing weight or not – is a balanced diet that won't deprive your body of the nutrients it needs. That means eating:

■ Lots of fruit and vegetables – at least 5 portions totalling 400g each day – to provide protective vitamins and minerals as well as dietary fibre. (Potatoes count as a carbohydrate, not a vegetable.)
■ Starchy carbohydrate foods like wholemeal pasta, brown rice and grainy breads, new potatoes, oats and other grains. These should be your main source of energy.
■ Lean meat, fish, poultry, eggs, beans, lentils, nuts and seeds to give you the protein, iron and zinc you need to nourish your body tissue.
■ Dairy foods like skimmed or semi-skimmed milk, cheese, low-fat yogurt or supplemented soya versions for the protein and calcium you need to maintain the structure of your skeleton.
■ A small amount of fat and sugar, for flavour and a well-deserved treat.

The Glycaemic Load or GL diet allows you to eat a variety of these foods without feeling hungry, which means that once you've lost that excess weight you'll be able to keep it off long-term.

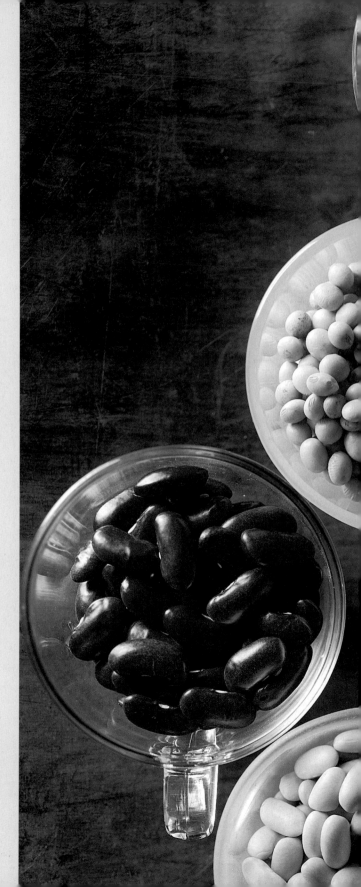

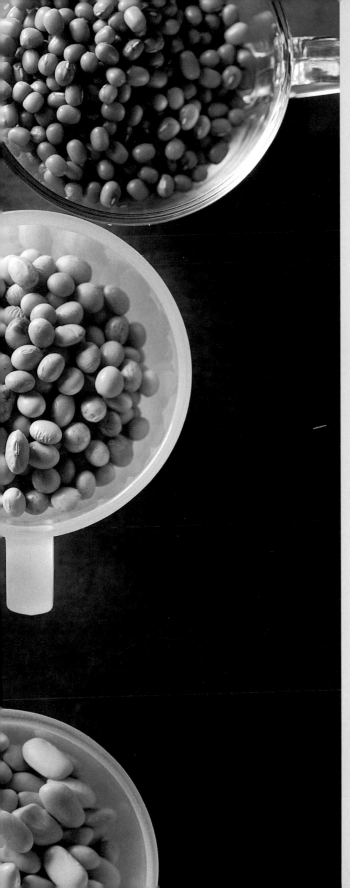

The origins of the GL diet

Researchers have found that not all carbohydrates are the same, which means that you can't group all the carbohydrate-containing foods together, as some diets do. Some carbohydrates are digested more slowly – they are said to have a low GI – which means that our blood sugar levels don't yo-yo up and down and we feel satisfied for longer. It is when our blood sugar dips that we feel hungry and prone to having a fit of the munchies.

So, basing a diet around carbohydrates with a low GL without eliminating any of the important food groups means we can lose weight while enjoying a wide range of foods and a balanced diet.

The Glycaemic Load or GL diet takes the Glycaemic Index a step further by taking into account average portion sizes and the number of carbs in an average portion. Foods are rated according to whether they are low, medium or high GL. As you will see later on, some foods with a high GI actually have a low GL rating.

FROM TOP TO BOTTOM: mung beans, soya beans, red kidney beans and flageolet beans

The role of carbohydrates

Carbohydrates should be our bodies's main source of energy (see page 14). Energy is required for all of the cells of the body such as the brain, nervous system, muscles and vital organ function.

Carbohydrates consist of sugars and starches. The sugars are further divided into the single sugars or monosaccharides. These are glucose, fructose (found in fruit) and galactose, for example. Then there are the disaccharides such as sucrose (table sugar), maltose and lactose, which is found in milk.

The starches or complex carbohydrates are made up of a number of glucose molecules joined together. They are found in breads, potatoes, pasta, rice, couscous, breakfast cereals, crispbreads and biscuits.

When carbohydrates are digested, the glucose in them is released and since glucose is in the form of very tiny molecules, it is quickly absorbed into our blood, causing a rapid rise in blood sugar.

Carbs and the GI
When it comes to the GI index (see page 12), glucose is said to have a GI of 100. All other foods are measured against this.

During digestion, the disaccharides such as sucrose are broken down into their component parts, so they take a little longer than glucose to be absorbed. Sucrose therefore has a medium GI.

Complex carbohydrates are also broken down during digestion to release glucose but the speed at which this happens depends on the structure of the starch. White and wholemeal breads are rapidly broken down and so have a high GI. However, if the bread contains less digestible items such as seeds, then it is broken down more slowly and will have a medium GI.

Oats and lentils contain fibres that slow down digestion, so they have a low GI. Pasta contains protein as it is made from a special wheat that slows down digestion. The shape of pasta also makes it less quickly digested.

The part played by insulin
In order for the glucose circulating in the blood to be used by our bodies for energy or stored as fat in our fat cells, a hormone called insulin, produced by the pancreas, must be secreted.

When we eat carbohydrates that are rapidly absorbed – those with a high GI – our blood sugar level rises very quickly and the pancreas secretes a lot of insulin in an attempt to remove this large amount of glucose from the blood and get it into the cells. Our blood sugar level falls quickly and we feel hungry again about two hours later.

However, if we eat carbohydrates with a low GI, our blood sugar level rises slowly and is maintained at a moderate level for some hours. The result? We don't have those hunger pangs so often and our bodies's secretion of insulin is moderated.

GI food summary

- High GI foods (70 and above) include glucose, white and wholemeal bread, white rice, mashed potatoes and watermelon.

- Medium GI foods (56–69) include sucrose, basmati rice, pineapple, beetroot and carrots.

- Low GI foods (55 and below) include oats, pasta, peas, lentils and nuts.

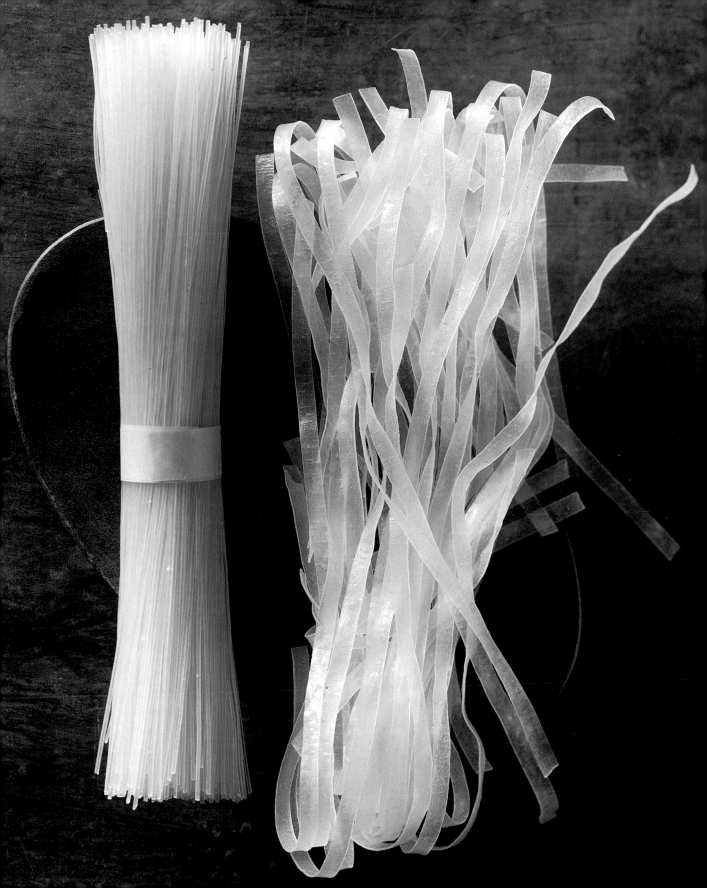

The Glycaemic Load

Work on the Glycaemic Index was started over three decades ago, in the 1970s, but it only became of interest to a wider public relatively recently. Now, though, knowledge about the Glycaemic Load – which is based on further research of the GI and the carbohydrate content of foods – means that it is possible to devise more useful dietary guidelines.

When foods were tested for their GI rating, it was done on the basis of feeding volunteers with food containing 50 grams of useable carbohydrates. Since the carb content of each food varies, the volunteers had to eat different amounts of food to get their 50 grams, so they'd need to eat a small amount of, say, pasta, and a large amount of, say, apple. Next, blood samples were taken from the volunteers over a period of time and their blood sugar was measured against their response when they were fed 50 grams of pure carb, i.e. glucose. Using these results, foods were assigned a number and the GI index was drawn up.

The problem with this is that the GI index doesn't give the whole picture because it doesn't reflect the amount of the food that people usually eat in one go nor the number of carbs in an average portion. For example, oatcakes have a low GI, but if you were to eat 4 of them, it would give a GL of 40 as oatcakes are mainly carbohydrate (you can see how GL is calculated opposite).

The same is true of a lot of high GI foods that, when eaten in normal portion sizes, turn out to be low GL, which means that there's a wider range of foods for you to choose from – and still lose weight.

How cooking and processing affect a food's GI
Cooking and processing usually soften and refines foods, resulting in a higher GI – the food is more rapidly digested and quickly raises the blood sugar level. In the past, there was less processing of foods, flour was wholegrain, and our grandparents ate more of the slowly digested

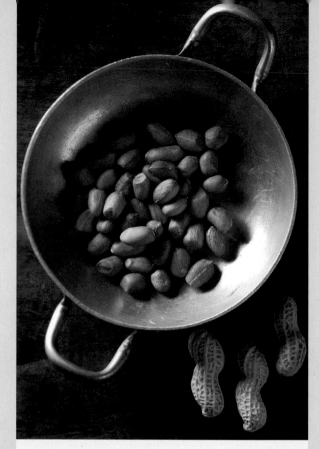

The GL range

Low	0–10
Medium	11–19
High	20 +

foods such as porridge oats, split peas, barley, dried beans and lentils. Much of today's food is highly refined and often pre-prepared to require minimal cooking.

Today's message is to slow down digestion by eating foods that are minimally processed, contain the original seeds and husks, are lightly cooked and kept chunky rather than puréed.

Calculating the GL

In this book, GL concepts lie behind all the recipes and meal ideas. There is no need to do any complicated calculations – though we show you here how the mathematics of calculating a food's GL works.

GL is calculated by multiplying the amount of carbohydrate contained in a normal-sized portion by the food's GI, then dividing the result by 100.

For example, **baked beans in tomato sauce** have an average GI of 48, which means they have a low GI.

A 135g portion contains 17g of carbohydrate (see page 24) so the GL is:

$$\frac{17 \times 48}{100} = 8.2, \text{ which is rounded down to 8}$$

Sugar (sucrose) has an average GI of 68, which means that it has a medium GI.

An average 10g serving (2 teaspoons) contains 10g of carbohydrate (see page 25), so the GL is:

$$\frac{10 \times 68}{100} = 6.8, \text{ which is rounded up to 7}$$

Wholemeal bread has an average GI of 77, which means it has a high GI.

An average portion of a large, thick slice (40g) contains 17g of carbohydrate (see page 23), so the GL is:

$$\frac{17 \times 77}{100} = 13.09, \text{ which is rounded down to 13}$$

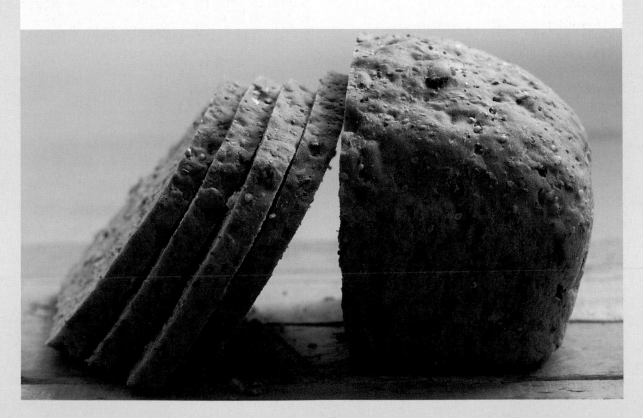

Losing weight

All the food and drink we consume provides fuel for our bodies's functions. Carbs are broken down mainly into glucose (page 10), which is the main fuel for our bodies. The energy a food contains is measured in calories (kcal).

An average woman requires 2,000 calories per day and a man 2,500 calories per day. To lose weight we need to reduce the number of calories we eat so that the body draws on our fat stores to get its energy. On average, to lose weight, we need to reduce our calorie intake each day by about 500 calories – so that means a total daily calorie intake of 1,500 calories for a woman and 2,000 calories for a man.

Limiting our intake to this amount of calories will give a slow steady weight loss of about 0.5–1kg (1–2lbs) per week. Dieters can more easily sustain this fairly modest calorie reduction than they can a severe reduction. It is also better for the body as it gives it a chance to adjust to the reduced calorie intake. Compare this with the shock to the body if you go on a diet that is almost a starvation diet and follow it with an overeating binge.

To help stimulate the weight loss you will achieve by reducing your intake by about 500 calories you also need to be more active and take exercise (see boxed text). If you do this, it will also help you to sustain your weight loss.

Carbohydrate energy
Ideally, about 50 per cent of the energy we need should be obtained from carbohydrates. If you are a woman who is trying to lose weight on a 1,500 calories a day diet, this means that you should get 750 calories from carbs. A man trying to lose weight should get 1,000 calories a day from carbs.

Each gram of carbohydrate provides 3.75 calories so a woman needs to eat 200g of carbs to get her 750 calories (750 calories divided by 3.75). A man needs to eat 267g of carbs to get his 1,000 calories (1,000 calories divided by 3.75).

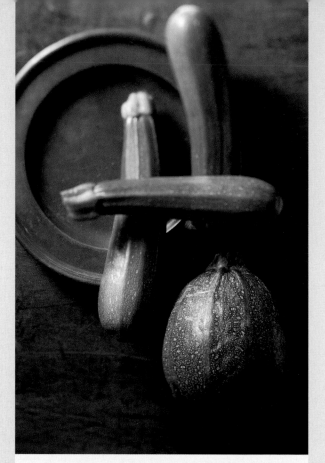

Activity and weight loss

Activity increases the amount of calories needed by the body as well as helping to tone up the muscles. It also helps to keep the joints supple and research has shown that it can help to prevent some types of cancer and coronary heart disease. Weight-bearing exercise can ward against osteoporosis, too.

Exercise also makes people feel less depressed and, combined with the more stable blood sugar levels supplied by the GL diet, can have an enormous effect on well being.

Ideally, you should take at least half an hour of exercise each day. Walking is easy. With just three ten-minute walks a day, you will quickly achieve the 10,000 steps a day that is the recommended amount.

The GL and weight loss

To keep our blood sugar at a stable and low level, about half of this carbohydrate needs to have a low GI (55 and below). However, as we now know from the work that's been done on the Glycaemic Load, some of the high GI carbs we eat are only eaten in small quantities and these can be balanced out by eating low GI carbs in bigger quantities. In addition, carbohydrate foods contain differing amounts of carbs.

Glycaemic Load principles take into account both the amount of carbs in your food and its GI. To apply GL to a diet, you need to find the GL you are allowed to eat each day. To do this, multiply the number of grams of carbs you are allowed by the permitted GI (55) and divide by 100. This gives a GL of 110 in the case of a woman wanting to lose weight and 147 for a man.

For optimum weight loss, your diet should have a lower GL than this; below 80 is often quoted as the figure to aim for on a very low GL diet.

To achieve this GL level you can eat a mixture of foods, combining those that have a low GI but which contain substantial amounts of carbs – for instance pasta and seeded bread – with foods that have a higher GI but which don't contain much carbohydrate, such as watermelon. Or a jacket potato with baked beans or porridge with a little sugar or honey. In other words, you can combine a range of foods to keep your overall GL low.

But to achieve weight loss, you also need to keep your calorie intake low. So, for example, while nuts and seeds have both a low GI and a low GL, they are high in calories, so eating them in large quantities will provide excess calories.

Whatever you eat, do so slowly, then your body has time to recognise the feeling of fullness that come about as the low GL foods take your blood sugar level to a moderate level then keep it there.

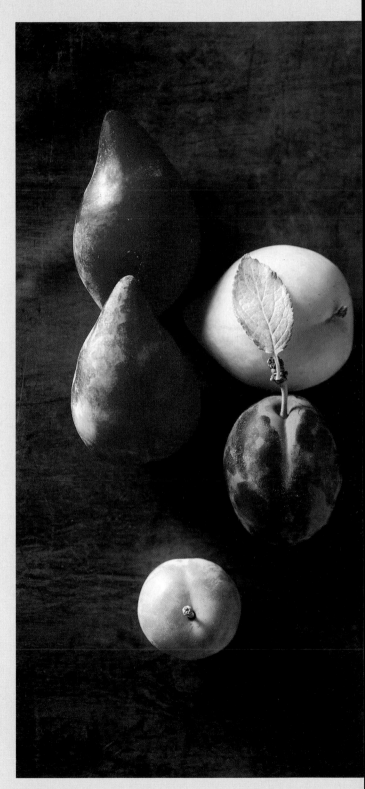

Zero-rated GL foods

We give the GI and GL ratings for a range of common foods on pages 23–25. However, fluids and certain foods that do not contain any carbohydrate have zero GI and GL.

Fluids

As we now know, fluids are an important part of a healthy diet as they ensure the correct fluid balance in the body. Fluids are needed for the body to function correctly, for digestive processes to occur, to keep the blood from becoming over-concentrated, for brain function and bowel health, to keep the kidneys working correctly and for skin hydration.

Ideally we should all drink 2 litres (about 8 cups or 6 mugs) of fluid a day. Water – either tap or bottled – is best and it has a GI and GL of 0. If you don't like plain water flavour it with a splash of fruit juice or by drinking herb teas. If you prefer tea or coffee, be aware that they contain caffeine, which acts as a diuretic and makes the body lose fluid, so make sure you drink your tea or coffee weak and always follow it with a glass of water.

You should try and avoid other drinks that contain caffeine such as colas as well as chocolate too.

Although alcohol has a GI of 0, it also acts as a diuretic as well as being a source of calories so if you are trying to lose weight, you should try to limit your intake.

Soft drinks sweetened with sugars and glucose often have high GI and GL levels so are to be avoided as they will give you a blood sugar surge. And of course, they contribute unwanted calories. Such drinks can be useful if you do a lot of sport and need an energy boost, but if you are tempted by them, try to have them with food to reduce the effects on your blood sugar levels.

Protein foods

Pure protein foods do not contain any carbohydrate so they all have a GL of 0. They include meats such as beef, lamb, pork and the offal from these such as liver and kidney. Poultry and game like chicken, turkey, guinea fowl and pheasant are also in this category as are all types of fish, shellfish as well as eggs and cheese.

However, as with all foods, these protein foods do provide calories so choose the very lean meats – those containing less than 10 per cent fat – such as lean pork, beef, lamb and poultry without skin.

You should also try to avoid too much hard cheese, which is very calorific, and use it just for flavour in sandwiches or cooking. Parmesan cheese and other mature cheeses have a strong flavour; a little goes a long way.

Eggs are a good source of protein, especially for vegetarians. Make sure that eggs are well cooked for pregnant women.

Suggested portion sizes for protein foods
- Meat – 100g raw weight
- Poultry or fish – 100–150g raw weight
- Cheese – 25g
- Eggs – 2 medium eggs

Fats

Fats do not contain any carbohydrate so they also have a GL of 0. But they are all high in calories so need to be limited and only used for flavour.

The monounsaturates found in olive oil and rapeseed oil, are regarded as the healthiest of the fats as they help to keep blood cholesterol levels low and are associated with lower rates of coronary heart disease.

Polyunsaturated fats found in soya oil, corn oil and sunflower oil also help to keep blood cholesterol levels low.

Saturated fats found in lard, hard cheese, butter and cream are associated with raised levels of harmful cholesterol and coronary heart disease.

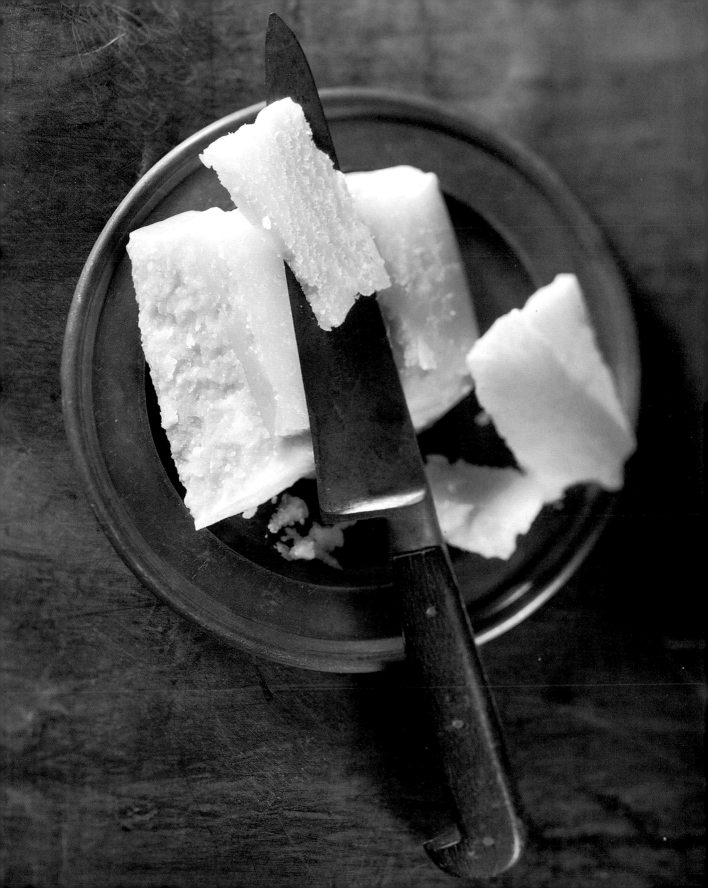

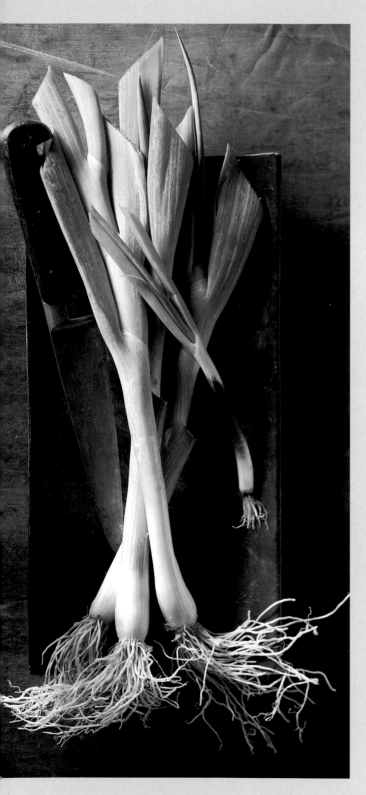

The benefits of the GL diet

■ As with the GI diet, you avoid the enormous highs and lows in your blood sugar levels. Children and teenagers are particularly affected by these extremes. Low blood sugar levels are often accompanied by hunger pangs which leave you craving for a sugar-rich snack.

■ You tend to feel satisfied for longer so the GL diet is easy to follow and easy to stick with and you aren't constantly craving a sugary fix.

■ Your energy levels will be more stable and you will feel less tired. After a couple of weeks following the GL diet, you will find that you have more energy and so you will be more active.

■ You may well also find that your moods improve, that you are better able to concentrate and that you are no longer prone to the irritability that sugar lows can cause.

■ Following a GL diet controls your blood sugar levels and your insulin response.

Why is the GL diet better than other diets?
■ It is based on simple, wholesome food that the whole family can enjoy.

■ There are no forbidden foods or restrictions on what you can eat, so it is less a diet, more a new way of eating. This means it is much easier to stick to than more prescriptive diets.

■ It is based on good scientific research so that after you have lost your excess weight, you can continue with this way of eating without any risk to your health.

■ It will give you a steady, healthy weight loss that will be easy to maintain.

How the GL diet can help with health problems

A low GL diet can be beneficial to almost anyone, whatever their age, but remember that toddlers need full-cream milk. You should also avoid giving them whole nuts and large seeds as they may choke on them. People who are ill should also not be given a low-calorie diet. Apart from these groups, a low GL diet can also help people with certain health problems.

■ It is low in fat and saturated fat so is beneficial if you suffer from high blood pressure, raised lipid and cholesterol levels and need a low-fat diet or a low-saturated fat diet.

■ If you have diabetes or insulin-resistance (syndrome X), you will benefit from reduced blood sugar levels and reduced insulin response.

■ It can help those with Polycystic Ovary Syndrome as well as women suffering from Pre-menstrual Syndrome.

■ It is high in dietary fibre so is helpful for anyone suffering from Irritable Bowel Syndrome (IBS).

■ The recipes are mainly low in sodium so they are ideal if you are on a low-salt diet.

The GL diet and exclusion diets
Nowadays many people have to follow diets that exclude certain foods such as milk, eggs and wheat. Other people have severe intolerances to nuts and seeds, while yet others have problems with foods such as yeast, onions and tomatoes.

If you are one of these, you will be pleased to know that some of the GL recipes in this book are nut- and seed-free, others contain no tomato, onion or garlic, and others are made without wheat, yeast or milk. Or you can make the recipes using the following alternatives:

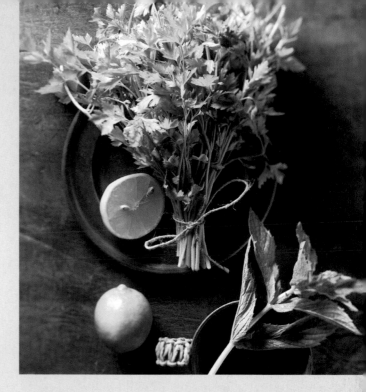

■ Toast branflakes, oatflakes and wheatgerm in a little olive oil to make a nut-free topping for salads.

■ Use soya milk (some lactose-intolerant people can also tolerate goat's milk) instead of cow's milk.

■ Try an egg replacer instead of eggs in the cake recipes (follow manufacturer's instructions).

■ Use wheat-free or gluten-free flour and add your own seed mixture to reduce the flour's overall GI and GL.

■ Try mushrooms, celeriac or fennel for flavour instead of onions and tomatoes.

■ Instead of adding salt to a dish, use fresh herbs, spices or lemon juice as seasoning.

Reducing the GL of a meal

It is relatively easy to reduce the overall GL of a meal by combining foods so that digestion is slowed down.

- Keep the portions of high GI foods small.
- Include large portions of very low GI and GL foods, for example low GL vegetables.
- Serve low and medium GL accompaniments such as brown pasta or basmati rice instead of white rice.
- Include low GI and GL fruits such as rhubarb, berries, cherries and grapefruit, either in the dish or as a dessert.
- Include extra oats in crumbles.
- Add seeds, oatbran and nuts to breakfast cereals, especially soya and linseed.
- Add lemon juice to a dish.
- Add beans to a dish.

Eating out on the GL diet

Eating out is a great pleasure and while restaurant food can contain more cream, salt and butter than home-cooked food, as long as you don't dine on rich dishes every day, you can enjoy your food without any feelings of guilt. However, there are a few low GL choices that you can make:

- Choose pasta and noodle dishes or small boiled potatoes in their skins rather than mashed or boiled potatoes and rice dishes.
- Ensure that you accompany your meat or fish dish with some low GL vegetables and salads.
- Eat fruit with ice cream rather than gateaux or pastries for dessert.
- Avoid creamy sauces, fried foods, breadcrumbs and butter.
- One glass of wine is fine, but bear in mind that alcohol provides extra calories.
- Remember that the occasional treat is fine – this is a diet for life and there is room to enjoy all foods as long as your overall diet is healthy.

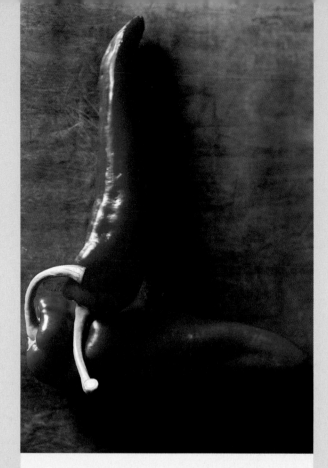

Low GL vegetables for your shopping basket

Aubergine	Leeks
Avocado	Lettuce
Beansprouts	Mangetout
Broccoli	Marrow
Brussels sprouts	Mushrooms
Cabbage	Mustard and cress
Cauliflower	Okra
Celery	Onions
Courgette	Peppers
Cucumber	Radishes
Curly kale	Spinach
Fennel	Spring greens
Green beans	Watercress

The GL diet and shopping

It is really easy to shop for a low GL diet. Many of the ingredients such as oats, pasta, seeds, dried fruit, barley, basmati rice and dried pulses are easy to find and relatively inexpensive. They will also keep in your storecupboard, so you will always be able to put together a low GL meal.

Health food shops offer an array of ingredients that are often not available in supermarkets so take a trip once in a while to stock up on unusual dried ingredients such as kamut, blue corn chips, spelt grains or buckwheat flour.

■ Don't be afraid to substitute. If a recipe calls for dried beans it's not a problem to replace one variety with another. The important thing is that you eat some beans. The same goes for red or black rice.

■ Buy seasonal low-GL vegetables. Not only are they likely to be cheaper, but they will also contain more nutrients and many will freeze well.

■ Packaged foods will usually have nutritional information on the labels and while most do not give GI/GL info, check the fat and calorie content.

■ Avoid foods that contain more than 10g of sugar, 20g of fat or 600mg of sodium per 100g.

■ Choose snacks or sandwiches that contain less than 300 kcal and main meals less than 500 kcal. If you think that this portion is too small, supplement it with extra vegetables or a salad.

Recipes in this book that you should be able to make from the storecupboard are:
■ One Pot Pasta with Potato, Green Beans and Rocket (page 79)

■ Butternut Squash Curry (page 77)

ABOVE RIGHT, FROM TOP TO BOTTOM:
hemp, linseed, sesame seeds

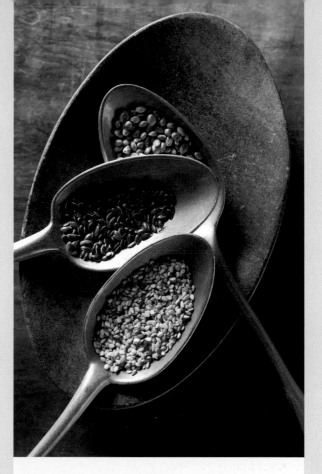

Storecupboard standbys

■ Tinned or dried lentils of all types, dried peas and beans and beans tinned in water
■ Pasta, preferably brown
■ Rice, preferably brown basmati
■ Oats
■ Couscous
■ Wholegrain or granary flour
■ Popcorn for popping
■ Dried skimmed milk
■ Reduced-fat coconut milk
■ A variety of spices and dried herbs
■ Reduced-salt or light soya sauce
■ Brown sugar and syrups
■ Dried fruits such as sultanas, apricots and figs (avoid dates as they have a high GI and GL)
■ Unsalted nuts
■ A selection of seeds
■ Low-salt stock cubes

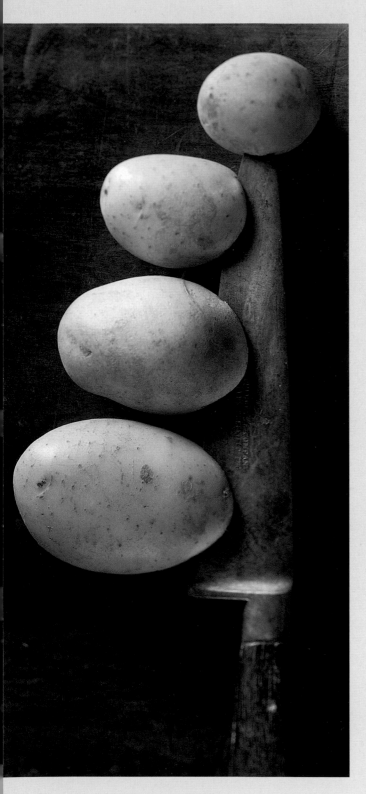

The GI and GL food table

The following tables give you information on the GI and GL of a range of foods, as well as their calorie (kcal) and carbohydrate content.

The figures in the tables are taken from various sources and it should be noted that the GI varies according to the variety of the fruit or vegetable, the recipe used by the manufacturer, the method of processing or cooking, and how finely foods are chopped (see page 12). As a result, these figures are intended for guidance only.

The GL is worked out per portion of food and the weight of the portion sizes we have assumed is shown in grams. For the sake of simplicity and to stay in line with the way nutritional information is presented on packaged food, we have also given the GL per 100g of the food.

Using the tables

Foods such as oatcakes have a low GI but are mainly carbohydrate and so have a high GL. This means that you should not eat them in excess.

Fruits such as watermelon and vegetables such as fresh broad beans, pumpkin and swede have a high GI but are mainly water and contain little carbohydrate, so have a low GL. This means that they can be included in your all-important daily five portions of fruit and vegetables.

THE GI AND GL FOOD TABLE

	GI	Cals (kcal)	Carbohydrate (g)	GL	Portion size (g)	Cals (kcal)	Carbohydrate (g)	GL
		PER 100g			**PER PORTION**			

BREADS, BREAKFAST CEREALS AND CEREALS

	GI	Cals (kcal)	Carbohydrate (g)	GL	Portion size (g)	Cals (kcal)	Carbohydrate (g)	GL
Kamut	53	140	22	12	40	56	9	5
Seeded breads e.g. soya and linseed bread	41	252	30	12	40	101	12	5
Quinoa	53	138	26	14	40	55	10	6
All-Bran	30	270	49	15	40	108	19	6
Oats (porridge, made with water)	42	46	8	3	180	83	14	6
Pearl barley, boiled	25	120	28	7	100	120	28	7
Pumpernickel (rye bread)	51	219	46	23	30	66	14	7
Bulgur, boiled	48	83	19	9	100	83	19	9
Oatcakes	54	412	63	34	30	124	19	10
Weetabix	69	352	76	52	20	70	15	10
Wholemeal rye bread	58	219	46	27	40	88	18	11
Crumpets	69	177	39	27	40	71	15	11
Malted fruit bread	47	295	65	31	35	103	23	11
Puffed wheat	80	321	67	54	20	64	13	11
Granary bread	61	237	47	29	40	95	19	12
Egg noodles, boiled	46	62	13	6	200	124	26	12
Brown bread	73	207	42	31	40	83	17	12
Wild rice, boiled	57	101	21	12	100	101	21	12
White spaghetti, boiled	37	104	22	8	150	156	33	12
Brown spaghetti, boiled	37	113	23	9	150	170	35	13
Vermicelli	35	86	24	8	150	129	36	13
Wholemeal bread	77	217	42	32	40	87	17	13
Macaroni, boiled	47	86	19	9	150	129	28	13
White bread	70	235	49	35	40	94	20	14
Hamburger buns	61	264	49	30	50	132	24	15
Branflakes	74	330	71	53	30	99	21	16
Buckwheat noodles (udon)	62	86	27	17	100	86	27	17
Croissants	67	373	43	29	60	224	26	17
Basmati rice	58	138	31	18	100	138	31	18
Pitta bread	57	255	55	31	60	153	33	19
Cornflakes	72	376	90	65	30	113	27	19
Crunchy nut cornflakes	72	408	92	66	30	122	27	20
Rice cakes	82	374	81	67	30	112	24	20
Muesli, Swiss	56	363	72	40	50	182	36	20
Arborio rice (risotto rice)	69	138	31	21	100	138	31	21
Couscous, boiled	65	112	23	15	150	168	35	22
Brown rice, boiled	70	141	32	22	100	141	32	22
Pancakes	67	302	35	23	110	332	38	26
Bagels	72	273	58	42	70	191	40	29
White rice, boiled	98	138	31	30	100	138	31	30
Baguettes	95	243	51	48	85	207	43	41

VEGETABLES AND PULSES

	GI	Cals (kcal)	Carbohydrate (g)	GL	Portion size (g)	Cals (kcal)	Carbohydrate (g)	GL
Onion	0	36	8	0	60	22	5	0
Lettuce, raw	1	14	2	0	20	3	0	0
Broccoli, boiled	1	24	1	0	80	19	1	0
Cucumber	1	10	2	0	60	6	1	0
Courgette, boiled	1	19	2	0	80	15	2	0
Avocado	1	190	2	0	100	190	2	0
Aubergine, raw	1	15	2	0	100	15	2	0
Aubergine, fried in corn oil	1	302	3	0	100	302	3	0

	PER 100g			PER PORTION			
GI	Cals (kcal)	Carbohydrate (g)	GL	Portion size (g)	Cals (kcal)	Carbohydrate (g)	GL
VEGETABLES AND PULSES cont.							
Green beans, raw	1	24	3	0	80	19	3	0
Green beans, boiled	1	25	3	0	80	20	2	0
Mangetout	1	302	3	0	100	302	3	0
Brussels sprouts, raw	1	42	4	0	80	34	3	0
Brussels sprouts, cooked	1	35	4	0	80	28	3	0
Beansprouts, raw	1	31	4	0	80	25	3	0
Soya beans, dried, boiled	20	141	5	1	80	113	4	1
Pumpkin, raw	75	13	2	2	80	10	2	1
Beetroot	64	36	8	5	40	14	3	2
Red lentils, dried, boiled	26	100	18	5	40	40	7	2
Green lentils, tinned, drained	48	64	10	5	40	26	4	2
Green lentils, dried, boiled	30	105	17	5	40	42	7	2
Swede, raw	72	24	5	4	80	19	4	3
Carrots, raw	55	35	8	4	80	28	6	3
Corn on the cob, boiled	48	66	12	6	80	53	9	4
Butter beans, tinned, drained	36	77	13	5	80	62	10	4
Chickpeas, dried, boiled	28	121	18	5	80	97	15	4
Kidney beans, dried, boiled	28	100	17	5	80	80	14	4
Kidney beans, tinned, drained	36	100	18	6	80	80	14	5
Broad beans, fresh	79	59	7	6	80	47	6	5
Sweetcorn kernels, boiled	48	111	20	9	80	89	16	8
Baked beans, reduced sugar and salt	48	73	13	6	135	99	17	8
Parsnips, boiled	97	66	13	13	80	53	10	10
Baked beans	48	84	15	7	135	113	20	10
Sweet potatoes, boiled	46	84	21	9	120	101	25	11
New potatoes, boiled in skins	69	66	15	11	100	66	15	11
Potatoes, mashed	86	57	14	12	100	57	14	12
Potatoes, peeled and boiled	101	72	17	17	100	72	17	17
Jacket potatoes	85	136	27	32	100	136	32	27
FRUITS							
Apricots, fresh	1	190	2	0	40	76	1	0
Rhubarb	1	7	1	0	140	10	1	0
Cherries	22	48	12	3	40	19	5	1
Raspberries	40	25	5	2	60	15	3	1
Plums	24	36	9	2	55	20	5	1
Apricots, dried	30	188	43	13	10	19	4	1
Blueberries	40	15	3	1	100	15	3	1
Blackberries	40	25	5	2	100	25	5	2
Strawberries	40	27	6	2	100	27	6	2
Kiwi fruit	53	49	11	6	60	29	6	3
Peaches, fresh	42	33	8	3	110	36	8	4
Oranges	42	37	9	4	120	44	10	4
Apples	38	47	12	4	100	47	12	4
Pineapple	66	41	10	7	80	33	8	5
Apricots, tinned in juice	64	34	8	5	100	34	8	5
Pears, fresh	38	40	10	4	150	60	15	6
Pears, tinned in juice	45	33	9	4	150	50	13	6
Grapefruit	25	30	7	2	340	102	23	6
Figs, dried	61	227	53	32	20	45	11	6
Bananas	52	91	14	7	100	91	14	7
Watermelon	72	31	7	5	150	47	11	8

	GI	PER 100g			PER PORTION			
		Cals (kcal)	Carbohydrate (g)	GL	Portion size (g)	Cals (kcal)	Carbohydrate (g)	GL
FRUITS cont.								
Peaches, tinned	57	55	14	8	100	55	14	8
Fruit cocktail, tinned in syrup	55	57	15	8	100	57	15	8
Grapes	53	60	15	8	100	60	15	8
Dates	103	270	68	70	15	41	10	11
Mangoes	51	57	14	7	150	86	21	11
SNACK FOODS AND DRINKS								
Olives	0	103	0	0	5	5	0	0
Pecans	10	689	6	1	25	172	1	0
Peanuts	14	563	13	2	25	141	3	0
Cashew nuts	22	611	19	4	25	153	5	1
Milk, skimmed	32	32	4	1	100	32	4	1
Yogurt, low fat, no sugar	14	47	7	1	150	71	11	1
Milk, whole	31	66	5	2	100	66	5	2
Milk, semi-skimmed	32	46	5	2	100	46	5	2
Yogurt, virtually fat free/diet, plain	20	54	8	2	150	81	12	2
Tofu desserts	115	261	2	2	125	326	3	3
Ice cream, low fat	50	119	14	7	50	60	7	3
Yogurt, low-fat, with sugar	31	78	8	2	150	117	12	4
Apple juice	40	38	10	4	100	38	10	4
Orange juice, unsweetened	53	36	9	5	100	36	9	5
Glucose sweets	100	375	100	100	5	19	5	5
Ice cream, full fat	61	177	17	10	50	89	9	5
Honey	70	288	76	53	10	29	8	5
Water biscuits	71	440	76	54	10	44	8	5
Digestive biscuits	59	455	69	40	15	68	10	6
Pretzels	83	381	79	66	10	38	8	7
Custard made with skimmed milk	35	104	16	6	120	125	19	7
Fruit yogurt, low fat	33	78	14	5	150	117	21	7
Sugar (sucrose)	68	394	100	68	10	39	10	7
Potato crisps	57	530	53	30	25	133	13	8
Wafer biscuits	77	537	66	51	15	81	10	8
Chocolate mousse	31	149	20	6	125	186	25	8
Chocolate mousse, low fat	37	123	18	7	125	154	23	8
Sultanas	56	275	69	39	25	69	17	10
Soya yogurt	50	72	13	7	150	108	20	10
Fruit bars	90	32	74	66	15	5	11	10
Raisins	64	272	69	44	25	68	17	11
Shortbread	64	509	63	41	30	153	19	12
Corn chips	42	459	58	24	50	230	29	12
Chocolate, milk	41	520	57	23	55	286	31	13
Chocolate, plain	41	510	64	26	55	281	35	14
Pastry, shortcrust	59	524	54	32	50	262	27	16
Cereal bars	72	419	65	47	35	147	23	16
Glucose-based drinks, e.g. sports drinks	74	60	16	12	200	120	32	24
Scones	92	364	54	49	50	182	27	25
Doughnuts	76	336	49	37	75	252	37	28
Waffles	76	334	40	30	150	501	59	45

About the recipes

All the recipes given here have a low GL so they are especially suitable if you want to lose weight.

■ We also give the calorie (kcal) content of each recipe and make a point of indicating which contain more than 300 calories. Where there is a range of portion sizes, the calculation is for the smallest number of portions. The calculations do not include serving suggestions.

■ As we have already seen (page 14), about half our energy needs to come from carbohydrates. So that you can ensure you are getting enough, we give the carb content of each recipe too. Where recipes have little carbohydrate in them (such as fish dishes), choose accompaniments from the lower GL starchy carbohydrate foods and vegetables.

■ The recommended maximum adult salt intake is 6g (1 teaspoon) a day, which equates to approximately 2,400mg of sodium. Many people watch their sodium intake because they have health problems such as high blood pressure. For this reason we give the sodium content of each recipe, which is generally under 500mg per portion. However, a few recipes have higher levels than this because they use ingredients such as ham, sausage, bacon, fish and tinned tomatoes. Try to balance out these dishes by using recipes with a lower sodium content.

■ Many people with raised cholesterol levels need to limit the amount of fat and saturated fat they eat. For this reason we also give the fat and saturated fat content of each recipe. In general, all the recipes have been devised to be low in fat.

■ For maximum GL benefit, do not peel fruit and vegetables unless the skin is especially tough. For the same reason, do not skin or seed tomatoes.

■ The recipes use medium eggs throughout.

RIGHT: Sprouted mung beans are high in vitamin C. To sprout your own, soak in cold water overnight, drain and store in a warm, dry place for 4 days.

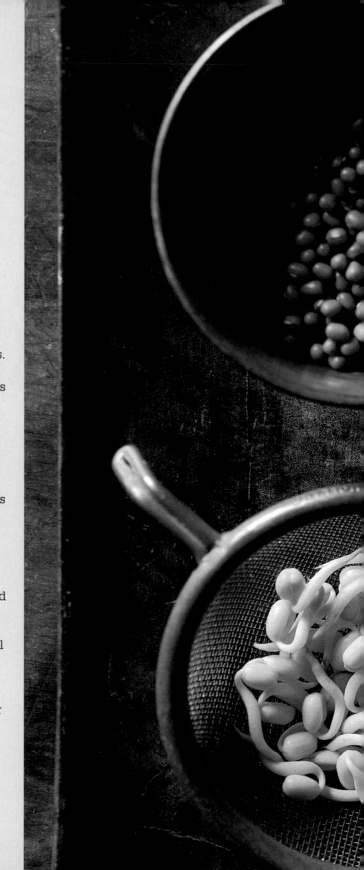

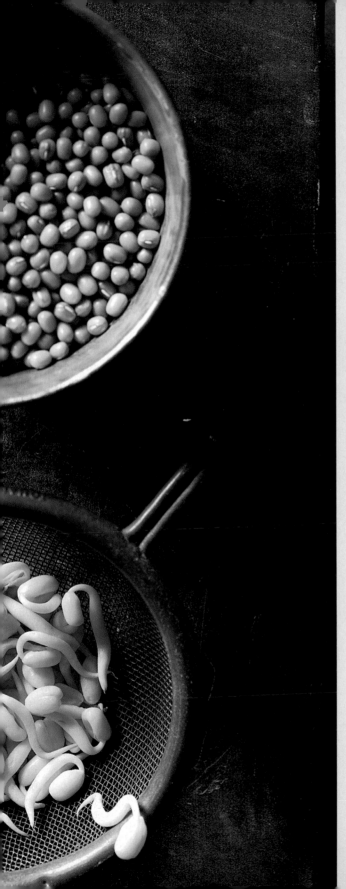

The GL diet made simple

In this book, GL concepts lie behind all the recipes and meal ideas. You will find that you can eat the foods recommended here and they will reduce the hunger pangs you usually feel when you're on a diet. What is more, the lower circulating levels of blood glucose in your body will mean that glucose is less likely to be stored in your fat cells – and that means less fat where you don't want it.

There is no need for you to do any complicated calculations – though you can see on page 13 how the mathematics of calculating a food's GL works. We have not given the GL of each recipe as the GL is affected by the type of ingredient you choose, as well as cooking method. It is also important to look at calorie and fat content if you want to lose weight. And as this is a way of eating that you can follow for life, it should not be about counting numbers, but rather being aware of the overall balance of your diet. So use these recipes with confidence and you will enjoy reduced blood sugar levels and sustained energy levels, without hunger pangs. This is the 'GL diet made simple'.

Be adventurous

You can always adapt the recipes by using different types of fish, seeds, grains, beans and fruits.

Not trying to lose weight?

The recipes in this book have been designed to contain less than 500 calories and to help people to lose weight. Those who are not overweight can eat larger portions of meal accompaniments such as bread and potatoes, and can have additional between-meal snacks.

Low GL meal ideas

Breakfast

This is the most important meal of the day as it literally breaks your overnight fast. It boosts your metabolism and increases your blood sugar. Breakfast also gives you an opportunity to eat foods that are high in calcium as well as others that are high in fibre. People who eat breakfast tend to be slimmer and also better able to concentrate.

If you are in a rush, you can grab an Energy Bar (page 44) as you go out of the door. They are also good for children. If you have more time, try the following:

■ Porridge, granola or a wholegrain cereal with skimmed milk and berries, dried fruit or honey

■ Grainy bread or toast with a thin spread of jam or peanut butter

■ Bowl of fresh fruit salad

■ Buckwheat Blinis (page 37)

■ Grilled sausages or lean back bacon with mushrooms or tomatoes

■ Eggs – poached, boiled, scrambled or omelette

■ Smoothies made with a selection of fruit and with added grains

Lunches and snack meals

It is also important to eat lunch. If you are out and about you can easily take sandwiches, salads or soups with you. The following ideas can also be used for buffet meals, picnics and children's lunches:

■ Raisin, Rosemary and Apple Soda Bread (page 38) may be frozen and means you can eat delicious fresh bread each day. You can also make or buy other types of bread for your lunches.

■ American Sweetcorn and Chilli Muffins (page 38) – excellent with soups and salad.

■ Onion, Cherry Tomato and Curd Cheese Pizza (page 40)

■ Soups such as the Minestrone Verde (page 79) or shop-bought lentil, bean and chunky vegetable soup

■ Salads such as the Greek-Style Village Salad (page 80)

■ Homemade salads with Dukkah (page 65)

■ Sandwiches made with seeded bread and filled with lean ham, chicken, tuna and salads

■ Seeded soda bread rolls (page 67) or granary rolls with fillings such as cottage cheese and salads

■ Wraps filled with salad and couscous

■ Prawn and Leek Pancakes (page 37)

■ Jacket potatoes filled with beans

Have fruit for dessert and as a change try a fruit salad; this travels easily in a plastic container.

Main meals

It is important to have a proper meal once a day rather than existing on just snacks. This book offers a range of main courses, which include meat, poultry and fish. There are also a number of recipes suitable for vegetarians. Some recipes are for one-pot dishes, which can be left to cook in a slow cooker or a pre-set oven while you are out. All the recipes provide substantial portions so no one need be left feeling hungry.

■ Meat such as chops, steaks or joints as well as fish fillets, which can be grilled or roasted and served with a salad or vegetables, plus baby new potatoes roasted or boiled in their skin or a basmati rice or pasta. The Vegetable Stir-Fry (page 82) and the Bashed Carrots with Assorted Seeds and Lemon (page 83) are quick to prepare and can accompany any simple meat or fish dish.

■ Leek Stew (page 86) or other types of stews and casserole

■ Thai Green Chicken Curry (page 108)

■ Seared Tuna (page 119)

■ Italian-Style Roast Monkfish Tail (page 124)

■ Fruity Beef Casserole (page 101)

Puddings and desserts

These give you the opportunity to include some fruit and milk in your diet. Obvious dessert choices are fruit and yogurts but you could also try the following:

■ Hazelnut Meringues (page 143)

■ Lemon Blancmange (page 143)

■ Cherry and Toasted Pine Nut Frozen Yogurt (page 145)

■ Hot Chocolate Soufflés (page 146)

■ Sparkling Elderflower Jellies (page 154)

■ Plum Oat Crumble (page 133)

Between-meal snacks

Fruit and pieces of vegetables make ideal between-meal snacks. You can also try the following:

■ Seeded Oat Thins (page 68) or other plain oat biscuits

■ Chocolate, Honey and Sesame Seed Popcorn (page 35) or plain popcorn

■ A small handful of seeds or nuts

■ A small pot (150g) of natural low-fat yogurt

■ Pieces of bread or pitta bread spread thinly with good-quality jam or peanut butter

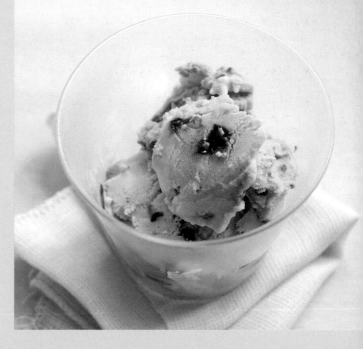

GL meal plans

The following meal plan ideas are for a variety of different situations – an average day; a day when you feel you need comfort food; a day when you have friends to stay; and a day when you are eating with children. Do not feel that you have to follow them slavishly; they are intended as inspiration.

Remember that:

- You can have 200ml of skimmed or semi-skimmed milk daily in tea and coffee.
- You should also drink 2 litres of water each day.
- You should use a minimum of butter or spread on bread. You may well find that with the delicious grainy breads and fillings suggested in this book, you do not need any other spread.

An average day

Breakfast
Glass of grapefruit juice (150ml)
2 slices of seeded or granary bread with a thin spread of plum jam

Mid-morning snack
Handful of grapes

Lunch
Cheese and Pear Wraps (page 92) and a large green salad made with cucumber, lettuce and cress
Low-fat Greek yogurt and raspberries

Mid-afternoon snack
Handful of raisins (25g)

Dinner
Vegetable Stir Fry (page 82) with basmati rice

Sparkling Elderflower Jelly (page 154)

Bedtime snack
Hot Mocha (page 150)

A day when you need comfort food

Breakfast
Bowl of Strawberry Porridge with Oatbran, Honey and Sunflower Seeds (page 35)

Mid-morning snack
Apple

Lunch
Chunky Beetroot Soup with Kidney Beans (page 80) served with a granary roll
Handful of cherries or grapes

Mid-afternoon snack
Low fat fromage frais (150g pot)

Dinner
Pork, Prune and Apple Hot Pot (page 111) served with green vegetables
Lemon Blancmange with Honeyed Blackberries (page 143)

Bedtime snack
Half portion of Chocolate, Honey and Sesame Seed Popcorn (page 35)

A day when you have friends to stay

Breakfast
Scrambled eggs on grilled field mushrooms with seeded toast (page 93)

Mid-morning snack
Slice of Walnut Bread (page 67)

Lunch
Dijon Mackerel with Scandinavian Potato Salad (page 127)
Baked Peaches with Brown Sugar and Almonds (page 135)

Mid-afternoon snack
Slice of Passion Cake (page 153)

Dinner
Mixed Grain Jambalaya (page 71)
Chocolate Semi-Freddo (page 146)

Bedtime snack
Dukkah (page 65)

Eating with children

■ If you have children under 5, avoid giving them nuts and small pieces of hard food as they can choke on them.
■ Toddlers up to 2 years need full-cream milk so don't give them skimmed or semi-skimmed.

Breakfast
Glass of unsweetened orange juice (150ml)
Bowl of low GL cereal and milk

Mid-morning snack
Nectarine or pear

Lunch
Onion, Cherry Tomato and Curd Cheese Pizza (page 40) with salad
Luxury Fruit Salad (page 134) with low-fat yogurt

Mid-afternoon snack
Apple

Dinner
Corned Beef Hash (page 111)
Plum Oat Crumble (page 133) with a small portion of vanilla ice cream

Bedtime snack
1 or 2 Seeded Oat Thins (page 68)

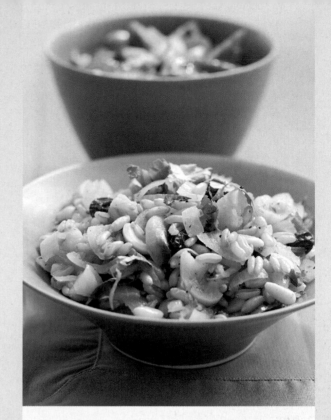

Entertaining

Many of the recipes in this book are easy to prepare which means that they are ideal for entertaining. And they are also great to serve to your guests since so many people nowadays are trying to avoid over-rich dishes containing cream and oil.

Try the following:
■ Iranian Fruit and Nut Pilaff (above and page 43)
■ Butternut Squash Curry with Coconut Milk (page 77) and brown basmati rice
■ Hot Chocolate Soufflés (page 146)
■ Sparkling Elderflower Jellies (page 154)

Spanish-style Spinach with Walnuts and Cumin (page 86), Braised Red Cabbage (page 85), Sweet Potato Mash with Dijon Mustard and Spring Onions (page 83) and Fiery Quinoa (page 44) are valuable additions to any simple meat or fish dish.

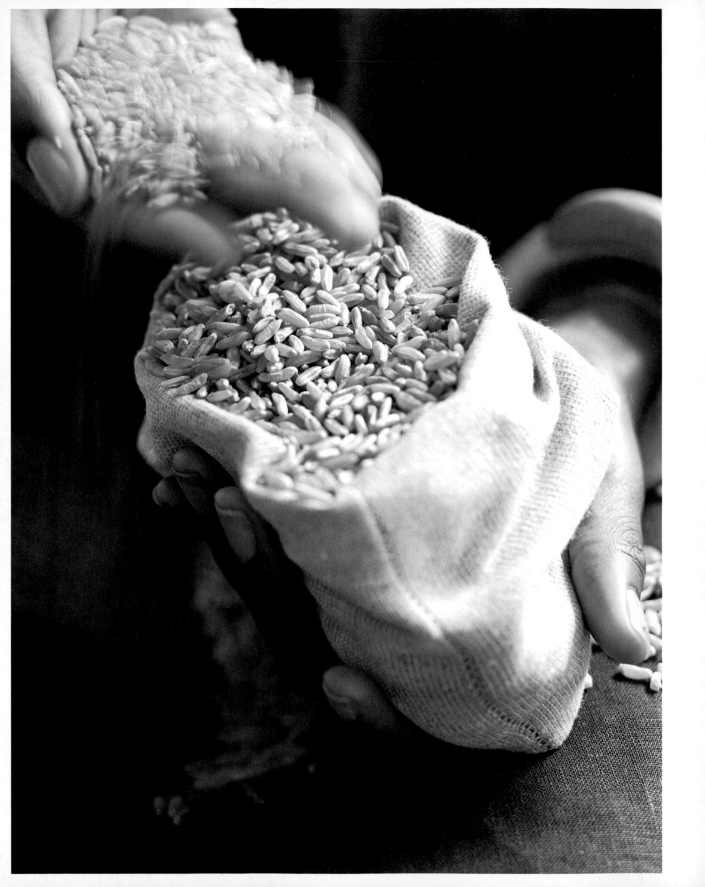

Grains and flours

About grains and flours

Grains and flours contain significant amounts of carbohydrate, which should be our main source of energy (see page 14).

Grains are the edible seeds of plants. Wholegrains are grains that have not had anything removed by processing and so they contain more fibre, iron, vitamin E and and B vitamins than refined grains. Wholegrain foods are obviously a better GL – and a healthier – choice than the refined ones.

Wheat

This is the major cereal in Britain and is used to make breads, couscous, cereals and pasta. Both white and wholemeal bread have a high GI but when seeds and wholegrains are added, the GI is reduced. If you do not like the seeded or granary breads then you should at least eat wholemeal bread, as it is a good source of fibre. Any flour you use should, ideally, be the wholegrain variety – the granary type with pieces of grain left in.

Another form of wholegrain wheat is bulgur. This is cracked wheat and the grains have been par-boiled then cooked to make them more digestible – again, it has a low GI. Couscous has a higher GI than bulgur wheat, so if you use it, mix it with low GI foods such as beans and vegetables.

Most of the pasta and noodles we eat in Britain are made from wheat. All pasta has a low GI (page 10), but it also contains substantial amounts of carbs, it has a medium GL. You can use the smaller varieties of pasta in milk puddings such as traditional macaroni pudding.

Wheat intolerance

If you have a wheat intolerance, use wheat-free flours, pastas and breads. Often these have a higher GI than the normal ones, so try making your own bread using wheat-free flour but add extra seeds.

Spelt flour sometimes causes confusion for those with a gluten intolerance. It does contain gluten as it is made from a traditional variety of wheat.

Corn (Maize)

Yellow maize contains the antioxidant beta-carotene. It is gluten-free, has a low GI and can be useful as a vegetable. If whole corncobs are not in season, use frozen or tinned corn instead (choose varieties without added sugar and salt).

Cornflour is normally finely ground and so has a higher GI than corn. If you prefer, you can use the more coarsely ground polenta instead for thickening casseroles and stews

Corn chips, sometimes called tortilla chips, make a useful snack, as does homemade popcorn. If you use a popcorn maker or a non-stick saucepan with a spray of oil, you will have a simple low-calorie nibble.

Rice

Rice is gluten-free. White rice and easy-cook rice both have a high GI while basmati rice has a medium GI. Wild rice, like buckwheat (see below), is also derived from a type of grass. It is also gluten-free and has a medium GI and GL.

The bran (husk) from whole rice is thought to have a cholesterol-lowering effect so choose the brown or unpolished varieties.

Oats

These have a low GI and GL and are the familiar oats we enjoy as a cereal. They can also be used in recipes to reduce the overall GI and GL.

Other cereals

Buckwheat is a type of grass and is gluten-free. It is often made into pasta and noodles and has a low GI, but medium GL.

Barley is a traditional British grain. It contains gluten, soluble fibre and has a low GL.

Quinoa is a gluten-free grain that usually comes from South America. Use rice as an alternative if you cannot find quinoa.

Strawberry Porridge with Oatbran, Honey and Sunflower Seeds

Here I have given quantities for 1 serving, so simply multiply up as necessary. You can vary the berries to suit your taste.

SERVES 1

50g whole rolled porridge oats
1 tablespoon oat bran
1 tablespoon sunflower seeds
1 tablespoon honey
75g ripe strawberries, hulled and
    roughly chopped
3–4 tablespoons semi-skimmed milk

1. Put the oats and oat bran in a small saucepan with 250ml cold water. Bring to a simmer then simmer for 5 minutes, stirring occasionally, until thickened. Add a little more water if you prefer a runnier porridge.

2. Transfer to a bowl, sprinkle with the sunflower seeds and drizzle with honey. Top with the strawberries and milk and serve at once.

Per portion: 370 kcal, 10g fat, 1.0g sat fat,
0.05g sodium, 64g carbohydrate

Chocolate, Honey and Sesame Seed Popcorn

This is a great snack, easy to make and children will love it. Good-quality dark chocolate has a low GI and contains vital antioxidants. Of course it contains quite a lot of calories, but it is beneficial in small quantities.

SERVES 2

50g popping corn
25g plain chocolate, minimum 70% cocoa solids,
    grated
1 tablespoon clear honey
1 tablespoon sesame seeds

1. Put the corn in a large pan and hold the lid on tightly. Set over a high heat and shake continuously from the point when the corn 'pops' until the popping subsides – about 5 minutes. Remove from the heat.

2. Add the remaining ingredients and toss well until evenly coated.

Per portion: 268 kcal, 17g fat, 3.5g sat fat,
0.004 sodium, 28g carbohydrate

Crunchy Breakfast Cereal

A healthy alternative to shop-bought products. Choose from the variety of fruit spreads available in health food shops to vary the final flavour slightly.

SERVES 4

100g whole rolled oat flakes
100g rye flakes
25g sesame seeds
25g brazil nuts, roughly chopped
25g whole almonds, roughly chopped
100g fruit spread (without added sugar)
50g plain bran cereal such as All-bran
2–3 bananas, to serve
100–150g berries of your choice, to serve
semi-skimmed milk or low-fat natural yogurt,
    to serve

1. Preheat the oven to 200°C/400°F/gas mark 6.

2. Combine the first five ingredients in a large roasting tin. Whisk the fruit spread with 4 tablespoons boiling water to make a smooth purée then stir through the cereals, seeds and nuts until well mixed. Spread out evenly.

3. Bake for 10 minutes, stir well and return to the oven for a further 10 minutes until golden. Leave to go cold then stir in the All-bran. Store in an airtight container.

4. Serve with roughly chopped banana, berries and milk or yogurt.

Per portion: 373 kcal, 15g fat, 2.0g sat fat, 0.14g sodium, 53g carbohydrate

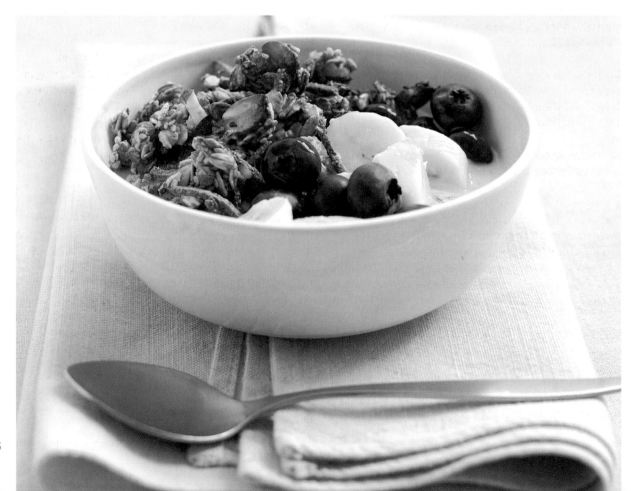

Buckwheat Blinis

It takes about an hour or so to make these but they are worth the wait! Serve with Greek Cherry Glyko (see page 149), honey or low-fat soft cheese. You can freeze any blini you don't need.

MAKES 12 LARGE OR ABOUT 50 SMALL BLINIS

1 sachet easy-blend dried yeast
1 teaspoon raw cane sugar
150g buckwheat flour
300ml semi-skimmed milk
75g strong white bread flour with kibbled grains
    of wheat and rye
150g 0% fat Greek yogurt
2 eggs, separated

1. Mix the yeast, sugar and buckwheat flour together. Lightly warm the milk in a pan (you should be able to hold your little finger in it) then beat it into the dry ingredients to form a smooth batter. Cover and leave to rise in a warm place for about 25 minutes.

2. Beat the bread flour, yogurt and egg yolks together until smooth and add the yeast mixture. Beat well then cover and leave in a warm place for 15 minutes.

3. Whisk the egg whites to soft peaks and fold into the batter until evenly combined.

4. Set a large non-stick frying pan over a medium heat. Lightly spray with oil and spoon on well-spaced ladlefuls of batter. Do this in batches of 2 or 3. Cook for 2–3 minutes until golden brown underneath then carefully turn and cook for 2–3 minutes on the other side until golden and springy to the touch.

5. Transfer to a wire rack lined with a clean tea towel. Continue until all the batter has been used up.

Per large blini: 102 kcal, 2g fat, 0.6g sat fat, 0.03g sodium, 17g carbohydrate

Prawn and Leek Pancakes

These dairy-free pancakes make a delicious snack. The batter can be made up to 8 hours in advance as long as it is kept covered in the fridge until required.

MAKES 18–20 (SERVES 4–6)

2 teaspoons olive oil
75g green part of leek or spring onion,
    finely chopped
75g plain flour
50g gram flour (page 50)
1 teaspoon baking powder
½ teaspoon paprika
freshly ground black pepper
4 tablespoons freshly chopped parsley
100g peeled prawns, chopped

1. Heat the oil in a small non-stick frying pan and cook the leeks over a low heat for 2–3 minutes until softened.

2. Combine the flours, baking powder and paprika with a generous amount of black pepper. Stir in the leeks, parsley and prawns then slowly stir in 250ml cold water to give a batter with the consistency of thick cream.
    You can use the batter straight away or leave for up to 8 hours in the fridge. You may need to add 1–2 tablespoons water if the mixture thickens during resting.

3. Heat a large non-stick frying pan over a medium heat and lightly spray it with oil. Pour on generous tablespoonfuls of the mixture spaced well apart, and spread them slightly – they should be about 5cm in diameter.

4. Cook for about 2 minutes on each side until golden and springy to the touch when gently pressed. Serve at once with wedges of lemon to squeeze.

Per portion (5 pancakes): 146 kcal, 2g fat, 0.3g sat fat, 0.17g sodium, 25g carbohydrate

American Sweetcorn and Chilli Muffins

Use lightly oiled non-stick muffin tins and not paper muffin cases for these, as this version without added fat is likely to stick to the paper. They may be frozen.

MAKES 9

175g coarse cornmeal or coarse polenta
175g strong brown bread flour with malted wheatgrains
1 tablespoon baking powder
1 teaspoon bicarbonate of soda
1 tablespoon dried oregano
½ teaspoon crushed dried chillies
½ teaspoon ground black pepper
2 spring onions, finely chopped
100g frozen sweetcorn kernels
1 medium egg
284ml buttermilk

1. Preheat the oven to 200°C/400°F/gas mark 6. Lightly oil 9 large muffin tins.

2. Mix all the dry ingredients together in a large bowl then stir in the spring onions and sweetcorn.

3. Beat the egg and buttermilk together and stir into the bowl. Mix well then divide between the prepared tins. Bake towards the top of the oven for about 25 minutes until risen and golden brown. Serve warm.

Per muffin: 160 kcal, 2g fat, 0.4g sat fat, 0.42g sodium, 30g carbohydrate

Raisin, Rosemary and Apple Soda Bread

There's no excuse for not having good bread in the house when you can make this in 15 minutes and eat it fresh from the oven! It also freezes well. For a more traditional look, shape each half of the mixture into a round and flatten to about 3cm. Mark into twelve wedges before baking.

MAKES 2 SMALL LOAVES (12 SLICES EACH)

500g strong brown bread flour with malted wheatgrains
175g strong white bread flour with kibbled grains of wheat and rye
2 teaspoons bicarbonate of soda
2 tablespoons freshly chopped rosemary leaves
100g raisins
1 medium cooking apple, cored and coarsely grated
2 x 284ml cartons buttermilk

1. Preheat the oven to 200°C/400°F/gas mark 6. Lightly butter 2 x 450g loaf tins.

2. Mix the flours with the bicarbonate of soda then stir in the rosemary and raisins. Stir in the grated apple and mix to a soft dough with the buttermilk.

3. Divide the dough, transfer to the prepared tins and cook for about 45 minutes until risen and crusty. Cool in the tins until the tins are cool enough to handle then transfer to wire racks.

4. Serve just warm or cold, or wrap in foil and store in a cool dry place. The bread will keep for 3–4 days but not much longer because of the apple content.

Per slice: 111 kcal, 1g fat, 0.1g sat fat, 0.09g sodium, 23g carbohydrate

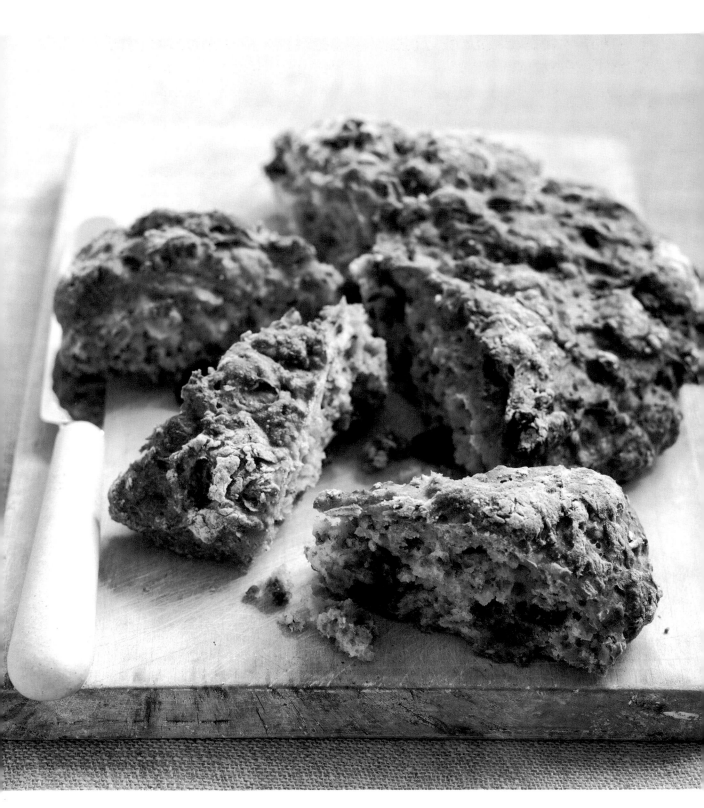

Onion, Cherry Tomato and Curd Cheese Pizza

MAKES 2 X 20CM PIZZAS (SERVES 2)

1 tablespoon olive oil
2 onions, peeled, halved and thinly sliced
2 garlic cloves, peeled and crushed
2 teaspoons fresh thyme leaves or freshly
   chopped rosemary leaves
2 balls (⅓ quantity) of Perfect Pizza Dough (see
   opposite)
250g cherry tomatoes, halved
100g soft curd cheese
freshly ground black pepper
fresh basil leaves, to garnish

1. Heat the oil and cook the onion for 5 minutes, adding 2 tablespoons water as necessary to prevent sticking. Stir in the garlic and half the thyme and cook over a medium heat until the onions are translucent – a further 5–10 minutes.

2. Preheat the oven to 220°C/425°F/gas mark 7. Put 2 baking trays in the oven to heat. If you have a pizza stone, now is the time to use it!

3. Take one ball of dough and knead on a lightly floured surface then roll to a 20cm round. Set it on a cold baking tray and spread half the onions on top. Arrange half the tomatoes, cut-side up on top and dot with half the cheese. Repeat with the second ball of dough to make another pizza. Sprinkle with the remaining thyme and plenty of pepper.

4. Transfer the pizzas to the preheated baking trays or simply set the cold trays on top of the preheated trays, and bake towards the top of the oven for 15–20 minutes until lightly risen and golden brown – check that the base of the pizza is cooked.
    Serve at once topped with a small handful of basil leaves.

Per pizza, including dough: 490 kcal, 15g fat, 2.3g sat fat, 0.85g sodium, 69g carbohydrate

Perfect Pizza Dough

The quantity of dough is sufficient for 6 x 20cm pizzas. It will keep in the fridge for 1–2 days or may be frozen for future use.

500g strong brown bread flour with malted
   wheatgrains
1 sachet easy-blend yeast
½ teaspoon salt
½ teaspoon freshly ground black pepper
1 teaspoon clear honey
1 tablespoon olive oil
250–300ml hand-hot water

1. Mix the dry ingredients in a large bowl. Make a well in the centre and add the honey, olive oil and 250ml water, then mix to a firm yet elastic dough. You may need to add the remaining water to achieve the correct consistency – the dough should not be sticky.

2. Transfer to a floured surface and knead for 10 minutes. If you have an electric mixer with a dough hook, then 5 minutes will be sufficient. Place the dough in a very lightly oiled large polythene bag and keep in a warm place for about 1 hour until doubled in size.

3. Punch the dough down and cut in six even-sized pieces. Shape each one into a smooth ball.

Per pizza base: 292 kcal, 5g fat, 1.3g sat fat, 0.83g sodium, 50g carbohydrate

Lemon Poppy Seed Rice

A delicious accompaniment to grilled meat or fish, as well as an ideal partner for Lamb Curry with Chick Peas and Spinach (page 105). Fresh curry leaves are available from Asian stores; dried leaves are sold in some supermarkets. This recipe will also freeze well.

SERVES 4

200g long-grain brown rice
pinch of ground turmeric
pared zest and juice of ½ small lemon
1 tablespoon vegetable oil
25g cashew nuts
1 tablespoon poppy seeds
1 green chilli, deseeded and finely chopped
12 curry leaves (optional)

1. Wash the rice thoroughly then drain. Pour 300ml boiling water from the kettle into a saucepan and add the rice and turmeric. Bring back to the boil, then cover and simmer for 15–20 minutes until the rice is just tender and the water has been absorbed.

2. Coarsely chop the lemon zest and keep to one side in the lemon juice.

3. Heat the oil and pan fry the cashew nuts for 1–2 minutes until lightly golden. Add the poppy seeds, chilli and curry leaves and stir for about 1 minute.

4. Stir in the rice, lemon zest and juice and heat through. Serve at once.

Per portion: 240 kcal, 9g fat, 1.4g sat fat, 0g sodium, 42g carbohydrate

Yogurt and Dill Bulgur

Bulgur is a wholegrain wheat and a good source of fibre. It is readily available in good supermarkets and health food shops. This is a Middle-Eastern dish traditionally eaten with pitta bread.

SERVES 4–6

15g unsalted butter
1 onion, peeled and finely chopped
1 large carrot, thinly sliced
1 stick celery, thinly sliced
1 leek, thinly sliced
1 teaspoon fresh thyme leaves
2 garlic cloves, peeled and chopped
750–900ml vegetable stock
250g bulgur
4 tablespoons 0% fat Greek yogurt
4 tablespoons freshly chopped dill
freshly ground black pepper

1. Melt the butter in a large saucepan over a low heat. Add the onion, carrot, celery, leek, thyme and garlic and cook, covered, for 10 minutes. Add 1–2 tablespoons stock if the vegetables start to stick.

2. Pour in 750ml stock and bring to the boil. Stir in the bulgur and cook for about 15 minutes until all the stock has been absorbed. Check after 10 minutes – you may need to add the rest of the stock.

3. Turn off the heat and allow the mixture to stand for 10 minutes. Fluff up the bulgur with a fork then fold in the yogurt, dill and pepper to taste.

Per portion: 311 kcal, 5g fat, 2.0g sat fat, 0.31g sodium, 57g carbohydrate

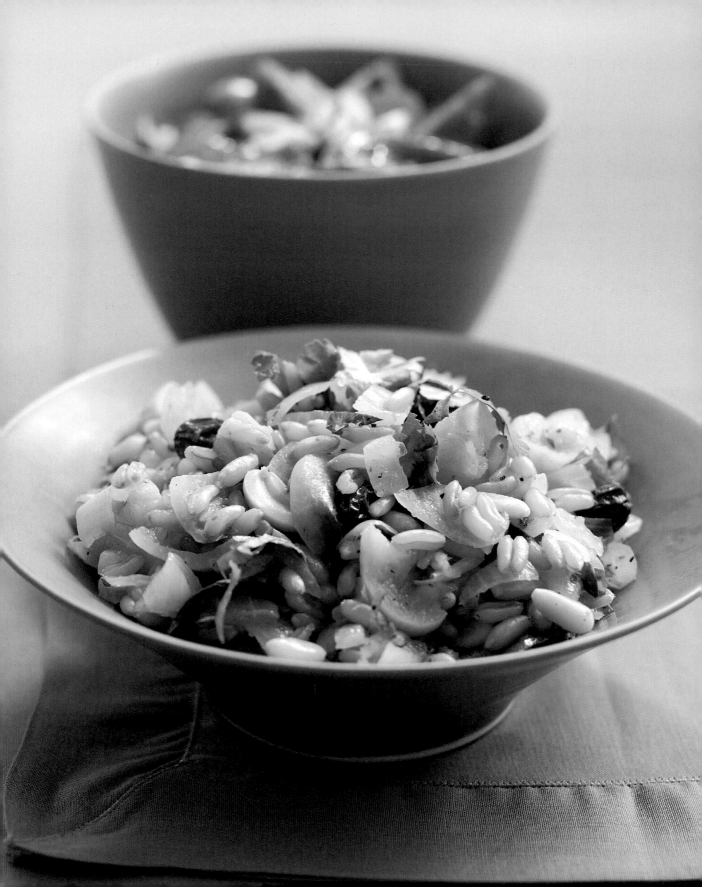

Iranian Fruit and Nut Pilaff

This would traditionally be made with rice but I like the 'nuttiness' of spelt or kamut grains, both found in large supermarkets and health food shops.

SERVES 4–6

250g spelt or kamut grains
1 tablespoon olive oil
4 onions, peeled and roughly chopped
50g raisins
75g dried peaches, chopped
finely grated zest of 2 oranges
25g raw cashew nuts
25g pine nuts or flaked almonds
600ml vegetable stock
2 tablespoons freshly chopped coriander
1 tablespoon freshly chopped flat-leaf parsley
freshly ground black pepper

1. Put the grains in a saucepan, cover with cold water and bring to the boil. Simmer for 15 minutes then drain thoroughly.

2. Preheat the oven to 180°C/350°F/gas mark 4.

3. Heat the oil in a flameproof casserole dish and cook the onion over a medium heat until softened, adding a tablespoon of water at a time, as necessary, to prevent sticking. Add the drained grains, raisins, peaches, orange zest and nuts and mix well. Stir in the stock and bring to a simmer.

4. Cover then bake for 30 minutes. Remove the lid, stir well and cook for a further 30 minutes until the grains are tender and most of the liquid has been absorbed. Season to taste with pepper and stir in the herbs.

5. Serve with a tomato and onion salad.

Per portion: 455 kcal, 12g fat, 1.5g sat fat, 0.32g sodium, 79g carbohydrate

Pumpkin Couscous

Barley couscous and pickled lemons are both available in Asian shops and some supermarkets.

SERVES 4

2 large onions, peeled, halved and thinly sliced
    lengthways
½ teaspoon freshly ground black pepper
½ teaspoon ground ginger
¼ teaspoon ground turmeric
2 pinches of saffron threads
250g carrots, cut in 4cm lengths
100g raisins
350g pumpkin, prepared weight, peeled and cut
    into 5cm pieces
410g tinned chick peas in water, drained
    and rinsed
50g pickled lemons, thinly sliced
350g barley couscous
1 tablespoon flaked almonds
1 tablespoon pumpkin seeds
lemon juice (optional)
2 tablespoon freshly chopped flat-leaf parsley
2 tablespoons freshly chopped mint

1. Put the onions and spices in a large saucepan with 900ml water and bring to a simmer. Cover and simmer for 30 minutes. Add the carrots and raisins and cook for a further 20 minutes. Add the pumpkin, chick peas and pickled lemon and simmer for a further 20 minutes.

2. Meanwhile pour the couscous into a large heatproof bowl and pour over 450ml boiling water from the kettle. Cover and leave for 4–5 minutes until all the water has been absorbed. Fluff the couscous with a fork.

3. Toast the almonds and pumpkin seeds in a dry non-stick frying pan. Stir into the couscous and season to taste with lemon juice. Stir in the herbs. Serve at once with the vegetable broth.

Per portion: 440 kcal, 6g fat, 0.6g sat fat, 0.18g sodium, 88g carbohydrate

Fiery Quinoa

Quinoa is a South American seed which can be used as a (gluten-free) alternative to rice or couscous. This is a tasty snack on its own with a green salad, or serve it as an accompaniment to grilled meats. Toasting the quinoa in a dry frying pan until it starts to pop enhances its flavour.

SERVES 4

250g quinoa
1 tablespoon olive oil
2 onions, peeled and chopped
3 garlic cloves, peeled and crushed
2 bay leaves
1 teaspoon dried crushed chillies
400g tinned chopped tomatoes
4 tablespoons freshly chopped parsley

1. Put the quinoa in a non-stick frying pan and dry-fry over a medium heat, stirring frequently until it starts to pop.

2. Meanwhile, heat the oil in a frying pan and sauté the onion until lightly golden. If it starts to stick, add 1–2 tablespoons cold water.

3. Add the garlic, bay leaves, chillies and tomatoes to the onions with an equal quantity of water and bring to a simmer. Stir in the quinoa. Cover and simmer for 20 minutes until all the liquid has been absorbed and the quinoa is tender. Stir in the parsley.

Per portion: 266 kcal, 6g fat, 0.7g sat fat, 0.09g sodium, 45g carbohydrate

Energy Bars

Wholesome bars of goodness, these make a great snack with a glass of semi-skimmed milk. Wholegrain crispy rice is available in some supermarkets and health food shops.

MAKES 12

25g desiccated coconut
150g ready-to-eat dried apricots
50g dried cherries, cranberries or blueberries
2 tablespoons vegetable oil
2 tablespoons crunchy peanut butter
3 tablespoons clear honey
1 teaspoon natural vanilla extract
100g whole rolled porridge oats
50g wholegrain crispy rice
50g raw cane soft brown sugar
25g sunflower seeds
½ teaspoon ground cinnamon
50g good-quality dark chocolate, minimum
    70% cocoa solids, melted (optional)

1. Preheat the oven to 180°C/350°F/gas mark 4. Spread the coconut on a baking tray and cook for about 10 minutes until lightly toasted.
    Alternatively, dry-fry in a non-stick frying pan.

2. Finely chop the apricots and cherries or whizz in a food-processor.

3. Put the oil, peanut butter and honey in a heatproof bowl in the oven for 1–2 minutes, or in the microwave on high for 30 seconds, just until they are easy to mix. Stir in the vanilla extract.

4. Mix all the ingredients except the chocolate until well combined then press firmly into a lightly oiled shallow 19cm square tin. Bake for 20 minutes then press lightly again. Leave to cool in the tin.

5. If wished, drizzle with melted chocolate and leave to set, then cut into twelve bars.

Per bar: 193 kcal, 8g fat, 2.5g sat fat, 0.03g sodium, 27g carbohydrate

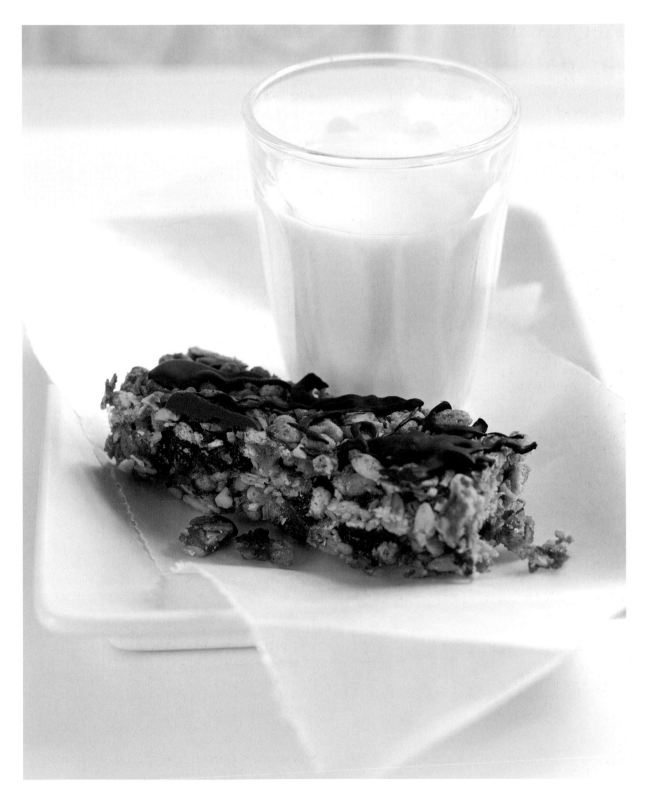

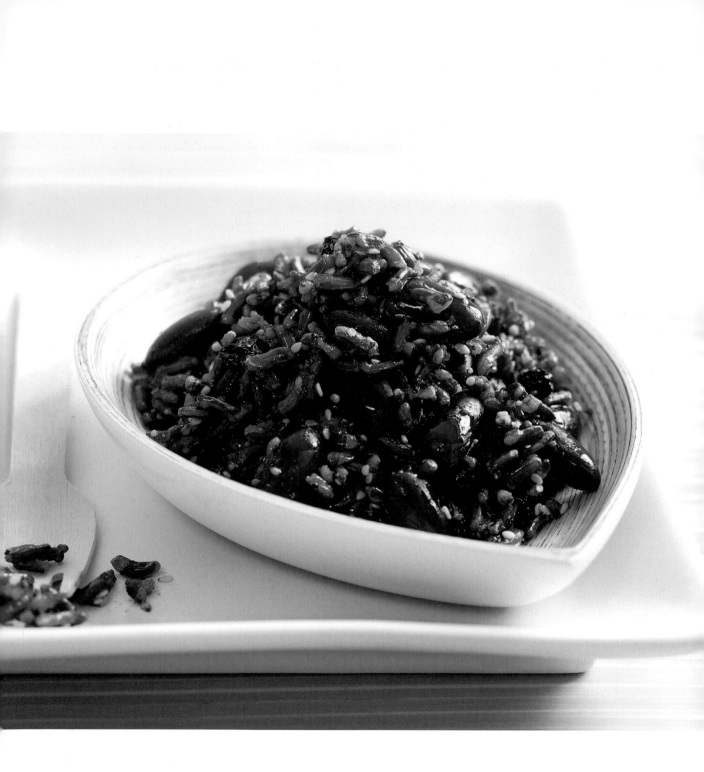

Red Rice and Kidney Bean Salad

Camargue red rice has a wonderful nutty and aromatic flavour so try it if you can. Otherwise substitute brown basmati rice and cook according to the pack instructions. Unless eating them straight away, always refrigerate rice salads as soon as you have prepared them and allow 30 minutes at room temperature before serving.

SERVES 6

175g Camargue red rice
75g dried blueberries (or currants)
410g tinned kidney beans in water, drained
1 tablespoon poppy seeds
1 tablespoon sesame seeds

DRESSING
1 tablespoon wholegrain mustard
1 tablespoon sherry vinegar
2 tablespoons olive oil (or sesame or sunflower oil)
2 tablespoons iced water
freshly ground black pepper

1. Whisk all the ingredients together for the dressing.

2. Cook the rice according to the pack instructions or until tender – 25–35 minutes. Drain well and transfer to a bowl. Add the blueberries and dressing and mix well. Leave to cool then add the rest of the ingredients and mix well. Cover and refrigerate until required.

Per portion: 225 kcal, 7g fat, 0.8g sat fat, 0.20g sodium, 38g carbohydrate

Oriental Basmati Rice with Beansprouts

This is a fragrant rice dish and a perfect companion for stir-fries. The beansprouts and peanuts will provide a satisfying texture.

SERVES 4

250g brown basmati rice
450ml vegetable stock
1 onion, peeled and chopped
1 tablespoon finely grated fresh ginger
1 star anise
150g beansprouts
1 teaspoon sesame oil
50g raw peanuts
8 spring onions, thinly sliced
1 tablespoon reduced-salt soy sauce

1. Wash the rice. Bring the stock to the boil in a large saucepan and add the rice, onion, ginger and star anise. Stir well, then cover and simmer for 15–20 minutes until the rice is tender and all the stock has been absorbed.

2. Meanwhile soak the beansprouts in cold water for 5 minutes then drain thoroughly. When the rice is cooked, stir in the beansprouts and set aside.

3. Heat the oil in a non-stick frying pan and fry the peanuts until lightly golden. Add the spring onions and stir until just wilted. Stir into the rice with the soy sauce and serve at once.

Per portion: 338 kcal, 8g fat, 1.3g sat fat, 0.42g sodium, 57g carbohydrate

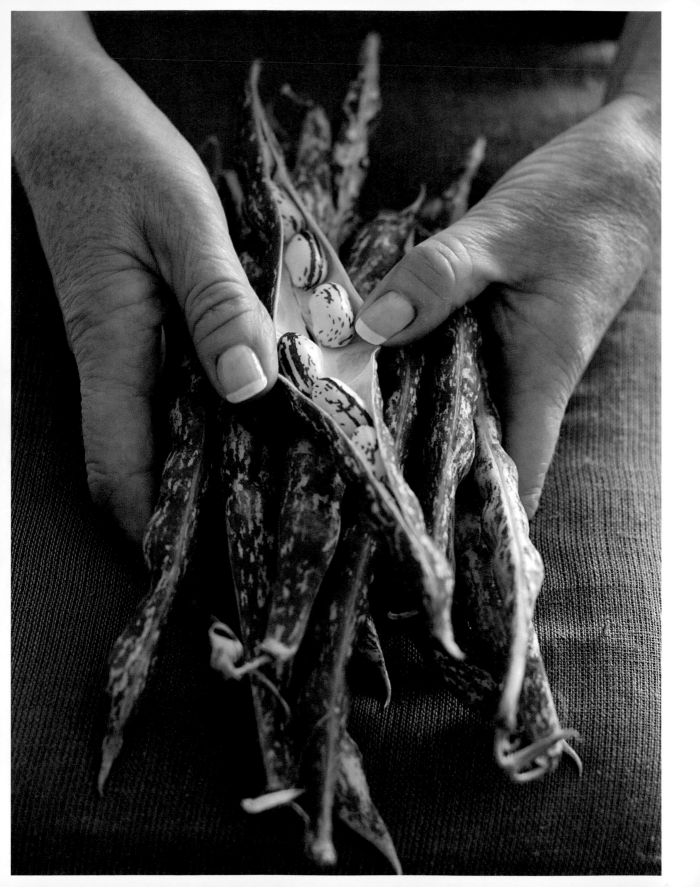

Pulses

About pulses

Pulses are part of the legume family that includes peas, beans and lentils. Many are dried to preserve them and this reduces their GI, which makes them a good choice, but they do need soaking and boiling before use.

For convenience, you can use tinned beans, peas, lentils and so on but, for the sake of your sodium intake, choose the varieties that have been tinned in water rather than in brine. If these are not available, drain thoroughly, then rinse them in a sieve before use under a running tap.

Beans

These are all low in fat and are a good source of fibre, protein, iron and zinc. All beans, and in particular soya beans, are also a source of plant oestrogens so they can be especially helpful for women. In countries where soya is a staple part of the diet (e.g. Japan), symptoms such as hot flushes in post-menopausal women are unknown.

Examples of beans are:

Adjuki beans	Cannellini beans
Baked beans	Flageolet beans
Black eye beans	Haricot beans
Borlotti beans	Red kidney beans
Butter beans	Soya beans

If you cannot find the type of bean specified for a recipe then it is perfectly acceptable to substitute another.

SOYA BEANS

Soya beans deserve a particular mention since, as well as the part they play in women's health (see above), their intake has been linked with heart health. The recommended daily intake is 25g of soya protein and soya beans are a good way of getting this amount.

Products such as soya milk, seeded bread containing soya, soya protein mince and soya meat alternatives provide other possible sources.

Peas

There are various types of pea – garden peas, sugar snap peas, mangetout, chick peas – and they are readily available fresh, frozen, tinned or dried. Fresh pea pods are less frequently found in the shops – you need to grow them yourself – but mangetout are a commonly available alternative.

Frozen peas are inexpensive and require no preparation. They contain all the goodness of fresh peas as well as retaining all the vitamin C.

Chick peas can be bought dried or, for convenience, tinned.

As with beans, it is the dried peas that have the lowest GI. It is easy to add these to casseroles and stews after soaking.

Chick-pea flour, also known as gram flour, is another option. It is readily available and is commonly used for making poppadoms. Poppadoms that can be heated in a microwave rather than those that are deep-fried make a good low-calorie, low GI snack.

Lentils

There are various types of lentils, all of which are interchangeable in these recipes and all of which have a low GI. You can buy them tinned but dried lentils only take about15 minutes to cook and so are a good low GI and GL storecupboard standby.

Use lentils instead of cornflour to thicken dishes such as casseroles and stews.

Pasta e Fagioli

This substantial soup/stew is a meal in itself and also freezes well. Serve with crusty seeded bread, if wished.

SERVES 4

1 tablespoon olive oil
4 spring onions, cut into 2cm pieces
2 garlic cloves, peeled and finely chopped
1 carrot, diced
2 potatoes, diced
1 celery stick, diced
230g tinned chopped tomatoes
1.2 litres chicken or vegetable stock
410g tinned borlotti beans in water, drained
   and rinsed
200g dried penne pasta
1 small hot red chilli, deseeded and finely
   chopped
8 basil leaves, roughly torn
freshly ground black pepper

1. Heat the oil in a large saucepan, add the onions and garlic and cook gently for 8–10 minutes until softened but not coloured. Add the diced vegetables and toss well. Stir in the chopped tomatoes and stock, bring to the boil, then simmer for 5 minutes. Add half the beans.

2. In a bowl, mash the remaining beans roughly then add to the stock with the pasta, chilli and basil.

3. Bring to the boil then simmer gently for a further 15 minutes, stirring from time to time to prevent the mixture sticking.

4. Season to taste with pepper.

Per portion: 409 kcal, 5g fat, 0.7g sat fat, 0.38g sodium, 77g carbohydrate

Real 'Baked' Beans

A far cry from the tins you buy and it's even better if the flavours are allowed to mellow for 24 hours. Freeze any you don't need.

SERVES 6

350g dried white haricot beans, soaked overnight
   and drained
1 teaspoon English mustard powder
2 tablespoons black treacle
3 tablespoons raw cane Molasses
   (or dark brown) sugar
4 tablespoons red wine vinegar
2 tablespoons tomato purée
230g tinned chopped tomatoes
1 onion, peeled and diced
175g back bacon, diced
1 bay leaf
freshly ground black pepper

1. Put the beans in a large saucepan and cover with cold water to 5cm above the beans. Bring to the boil then simmer, partially covered, until the beans are tender, about 1¼ hours.

2. Meanwhile, blend the mustard powder with a little water to make a thin paste, then combine with the treacle, sugar, vinegar, tomato purée and tomatoes. Set aside.

3. Fry the onion and bacon in a dry non-stick frying pan for 8–10 minutes until the onion is softened but not coloured.

4. Drain the beans and return to the pan. Add the reserved flavouring liquid, the onion mixture, the bay leaf and plenty of pepper and bring to a simmer. Simmer, uncovered, for 45–60 minutes until most of the liquid has evaporated. Serve piping hot with crusty bread.

Per portion: 337 kcal, 8g fat, 2.6g sat fat, 0.48g sodium, 51g carbohydrate

Houmous with a Twist

Try serving this with chunks of cucumber and carrot as an alternative to bread. Or make pitta crisps by cutting wholemeal pitta bread in small triangles, then in half horizontally and drying out in a warm oven at 180°C/350°F/gas mark 4 for 10–15 minutes until crisp.

SERVES 4

410g tinned chick peas in water, drained and
    water reserved
2 tablespoons tahini
2 garlic cloves, peeled and crushed
3 tablespoons lemon juice
1 tablespoon olive oil
paprika, to taste
1 roasted red pepper, finely diced (available
    in tins or jars, or roast your own, see page 61)
15g sunflower seeds
15g flaked almonds or pine nuts, toasted
wholemeal pitta bread, to serve
black olives (optional), to serve

1. Place the chick peas in a food-processor with 3 tablespoons of the reserved water, the tahini and garlic. Blend until fairly smooth.

2. Add the lemon juice followed by the oil. Season with paprika, to taste.

3. Gently fold in the roasted red pepper, sunflower seeds and almonds.

4. Serve with warm wholemeal pitta bread and garnish with black olives.

Per portion: 238 kcal, 16g fat, 0.8g sat fat, 0.07g sodium, 15g carbohydrate

Pea Guacamole

A perfect storecupboard starter that can be made on short notice. Serve it with corn chips or use as a topping for grilled salmon.

SERVES 4

250g frozen peas, cooked and well drained
1 tablespoon lime juice
1 tablespoon fresh coriander leaves
1 red chilli, deseeded and diced
2 tablespoons 0% fat Greek yogurt
¼ teaspoon ground cumin
¼ teaspoon ground coriander
¼ teaspoon freshly ground black pepper
1 plum tomato, chopped
¼ small red onion, peeled and finely chopped

1. Put all the ingredients except the tomato and onion in a food-processor and pulse until fairly smooth.

2. Stir in the tomato and onion and serve with corn chips.

VARIATION
Replace the peas with sweetcorn.

Per portion: 62 kcal, 1g fat, 0.2g sat fat, 0g sodium, 8g carbohydrate

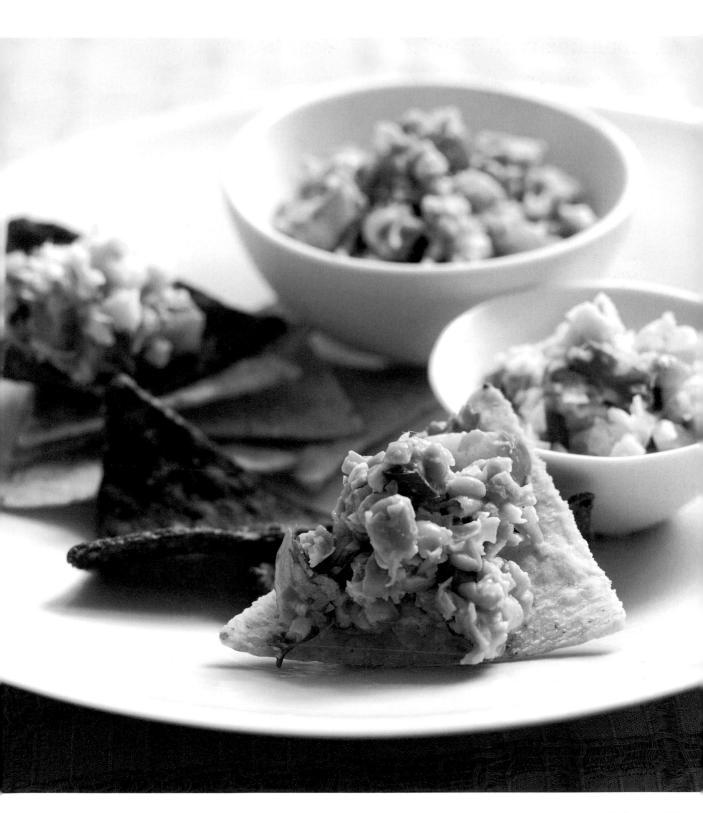

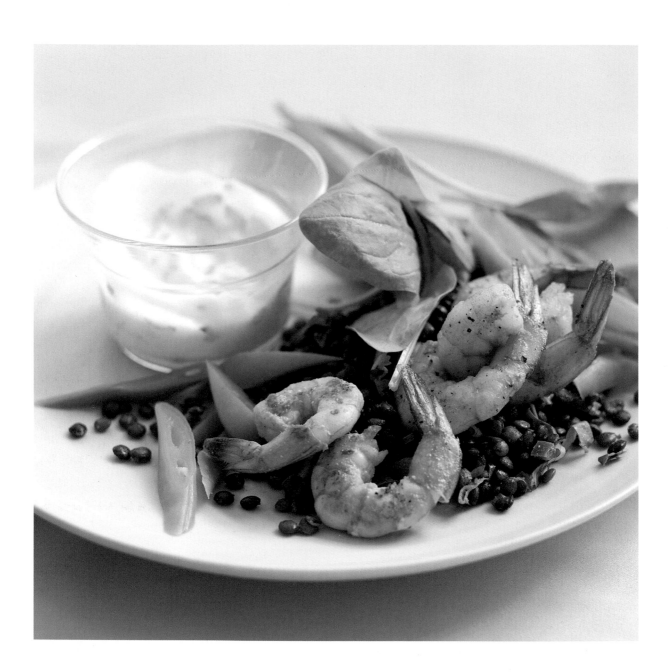

Spiced Lentil Salad with Prawns and Mint Yogurt

A wonderful combination of flavours with simple preparation makes a great dish for entertaining.

SERVES 4

200g Puy lentils, cooked until just tender, drained and kept warm
2 spring onions, thinly sliced
2 tablespoons red wine vinegar
1 green chilli, deseeded and finely chopped
1 teaspoon ground coriander
1 teaspoon ground cumin
4 tablespoons freshly chopped coriander
2 tablespoons olive oil
½ teaspoon ground turmeric
20 raw prawns (about 200g), peeled and deveined, tails intact
2 handfuls (about 50g) baby spinach leaves
100g green beans, blanched
freshly ground black pepper

MINT YOGURT DIP
300g 0% fat Greek yogurt
2 teaspoons fish sauce (nam pla)
2 tablespoons fresh lime juice
4 tablespoons freshly chopped mint

1. In a bowl, mix the warm lentils, spring onions, vinegar, chilli, ground spices, coriander and 1 tablespoon oil. Add pepper and set aside.

2. Mix the remaining oil, turmeric and some pepper in another bowl and turn the prawns in the mixture to coat them. Preheat a non-stick frying pan. Cook the for 3 minutes, turning once, until opaque.

3. Mix the dip ingredients together.

4. Divide the lentils between four plates, top with baby spinach leaves, green beans and prawns and serve with the dip.

Per portion: 290 kcal, 7g fat, 1.0g sat fat, 0.23g sodium, 29g carbohydrate

Kamut with Peas, Spring Onions and Mint

An easy meal from the storecupboard. You can experiment with different sorts of pasta. Here I've used kamut tagliatelle – a ribbon pasta made from an old-fashioned type of wheat – but traditional tagliatelle is fine.

SERVES 4

350g kamut tagliatelle (see above)
15g unsalted butter
6 spring onions, sliced
250g frozen peas
3 tablespoons freshly chopped mint
a handful of sorrel leaves, shredded
    (or watercress or rocket)
50g freshly grated Parmesan
freshly ground black pepper

1. Cook the kamut in boiling water for 12–15 minutes. Drain thoroughly.

2. Meanwhile, put the butter, spring onions, peas and 125ml water in a saucepan and simmer, covered, for 7–8 minutes until tender. Fold in the mint and sorrel just to wilt it.

3. Toss the pea mixture with the pasta, Parmesan and plenty of black pepper and serve at once.

Per portion: 431 kcal, 9g fat, 4.8g sat fat, 0.11g sodium, 73g carbohydrate

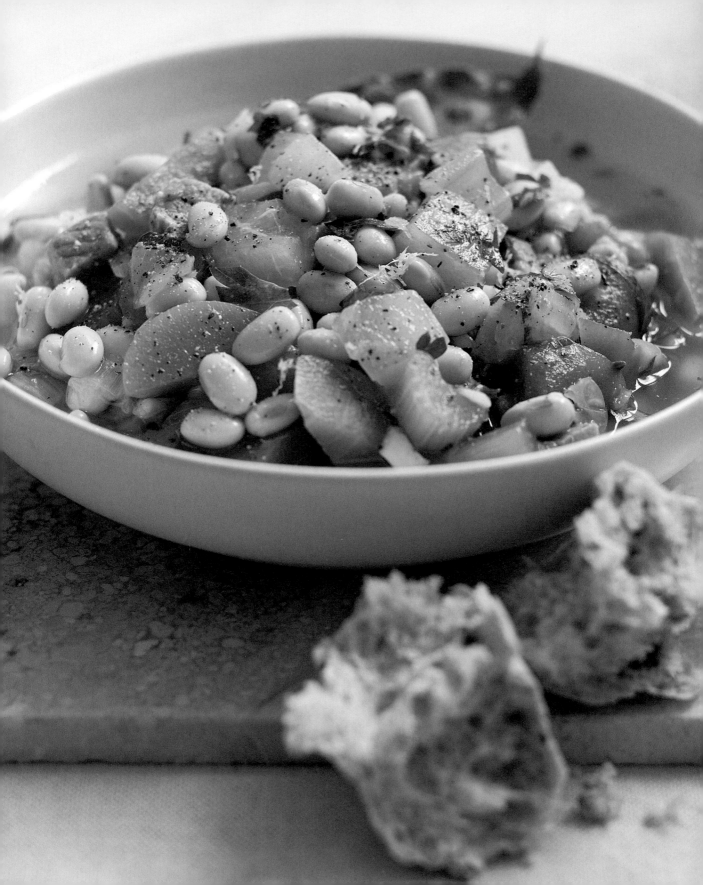

Soya Bean Stew with Gremolata

You need to soak the beans overnight for this recipe. Once made and cooled, the stew will keep in the fridge for up to 2 days. Re-heat as necessary and add the gremolata (a parsley and lemon-based dressing) just before serving.

SERVES 4–6

250g soya beans, soaked overnight
2 large onions, peeled and roughly chopped
2 garlic cloves, peeled and chopped
200g raw lean gammon, cubed
a few sprigs of fresh thyme
a few sprigs of fresh rosemary
2 bay leaves
1½ litres vegetable stock or water
4 carrots, cut into chunks
4 sticks celery, cut into chunks
1 large turnip – roughly 250g – cut into chunks
¼ medium swede – roughly 200g – cut into chunks
freshly ground black pepper

GREMOLATA
4 tablespoons freshly chopped parsley
finely grated zest of 1 lemon
2 garlic cloves, peeled and finely chopped

1. Drain the soaked beans and rinse. Put them in a large saucepan and cover with cold water. Bring to the boil then simmer for 15 minutes. Drain once more.

2. Place the beans in a large flameproof casserole or saucepan and add half the onion, the garlic, ham and herbs and cover with the stock. Bring to a simmer then simmer for 1 hour. Add all the remaining ingredients and simmer for a further 1 hour until the beans are tender. Discard any herb stalks then season to taste.

3. Combine the ingredients for the gremolata and stir in just before serving.

Per portion: 411 kcal, 17g fat, 2.8g sat fat, 0.80g sodium, 33g carbohydrate

Savoury Mince with Lentils

Mince is so versatile and easy to use and combining it with lentils reduces its GI as well as giving added interest and texture. This savoury dish is good as a simple meal with vegetables but also great spooned over a jacket potato – either a sweet potato or a traditional one – or with pasta. This recipe is also good for freezing.

SERVES 6

400g very lean minced beef
1 onion, peeled and chopped
1 teaspoon English mustard powder
½ teaspoon freshly ground black pepper
2 tablespoons Worcestershire sauce
2 tablespoons tomato purée
400g tinned chopped tomatoes
200g green lentils, rinsed
2 tablespoons freshly chopped parsley
2 tablespoons freshly chopped chives

1. Put the beef and onion in a large non-stick frying pan and cook over a medium heat, stirring frequently until they are well browned.

2. Add the mustard, pepper, Worcestershire sauce and tomato purée and stir well. Add the tomatoes with 1 tin water and bring to a simmer.

3. Stir in the lentils, then cover and simmer for 30 minutes until well cooked and reduced to a rich sauce. Add the chopped herbs just before serving.

Per portion: 217 kcal, 4g fat, 1.4g sat fat, 0.09g sodium, 22g carbohydrate

Lentil and Coriander Burgers

These are really satisfying veggie burgers. Make sure you cook the lentils thoroughly so that they will mash sufficiently to bind the mixture together.

MAKES 8–12/SERVES 4

1 tablespoon olive oil
1 large onion, peeled and finely chopped
2 carrots, finely chopped
1 celery stalk, finely chopped
2 garlic cloves, peeled and crushed
1 large red chilli, deseeded and finely chopped
225g Puy lentils, cooked until tender then
     thoroughly drained
1 teaspoon ground cumin
1 teaspoon ground coriander
3 tablespoons freshly chopped coriander
3 tablespoons freshly chopped parsley
1 egg yolk
1 tablespoon wholegrain flour
freshly ground black pepper
cornflour, for shaping

1. Heat the oil and fry the onion, carrots, celery, garlic and chilli for 8–10 minutes until softened but not coloured. Remove from the heat and allow to cool.

2. Place the cooked vegetables in a food-processor with the lentils, spices, herbs, egg yolk and flour. Pulse until the mixture binds and holds together. Season generously with pepper.

3. With floured hands, shape into 8–12 patties.

4. Preheat the grill to maximum and cook the burgers until crispy on both sides, 6–8 minutes. Handle the burgers carefully as they can be very delicate.

5. Serve with a yogurt dip and a leaf salad.

Per portion: 271 kcal, 6g fat, 1.0g sat fat, 0.03g sodium, 41g carbohydrate

Traditional Meatball Stew

MAKES 20–24/SERVES 4

1 tablespoon olive oil
1 onion, peeled and roughly chopped
1 stick celery and 1 large carrot, cut in 2cm pieces
1 garlic clove, peeled and finely chopped
½ tablespoon fresh thyme leaves
1 bay leaf
1 leek, halved lengthways, cut into 2cm pieces
100g piece of lean raw ham, cut into 1cm pieces
1 litre chicken stock
50g millet seeds, dry-fried until they pop
400g tinned pinto beans in water, drained, rinsed
MEATBALLS
200g minced pork
400g tinned haricot beans in water, drained,
     rinsed (use ¼ and reserve the rest for the stew)
25g dried apple, finely chopped
1 tablespoon freshly grated root ginger
1 shallot, finely chopped
8 tablespoons multi-seeded fresh breadcrumbs
1 medium egg white, lightly beaten
1 tablespoon tomato purée
½ teaspoon ground nutmeg
1 tablespoon chopped parsley
1 tablespoon snipped chives
1 tablespoon olive oil

1. Heat the oil, add the next six ingredients and cook over a medium heat for 10 minutes. Add the leek, ham and chicken stock, cover and cook gently for 45 minutes, skimming occasionally. Add the millet, pinto beans and reserved haricot beans and cook for a further 30 minutes. Season with pepper.

2. Meanwhile, make the meatballs. Combine all the ingredients except the oil. Season with pepper, then shape into 20–24 balls, about 2.5cm diameter. Heat the oil in a frying pan and fry in batches until well browned. Pop them into the stew and simmer, covered, for a further 20 minutes. Season and serve piping hot in bowls.

Per portion: 466 kcal, 11g fat, 2.1g sat fat, 1.08g sodium, 64g carbohydrate

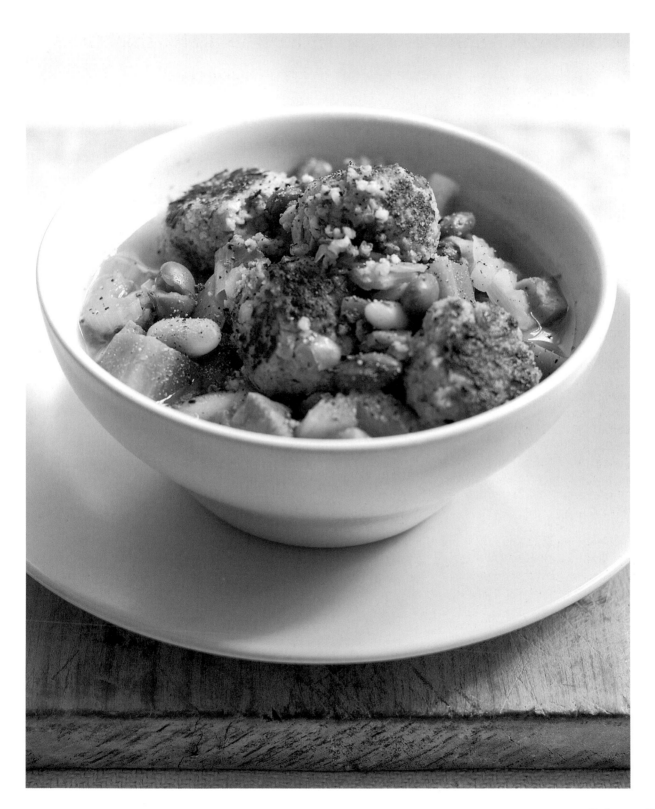

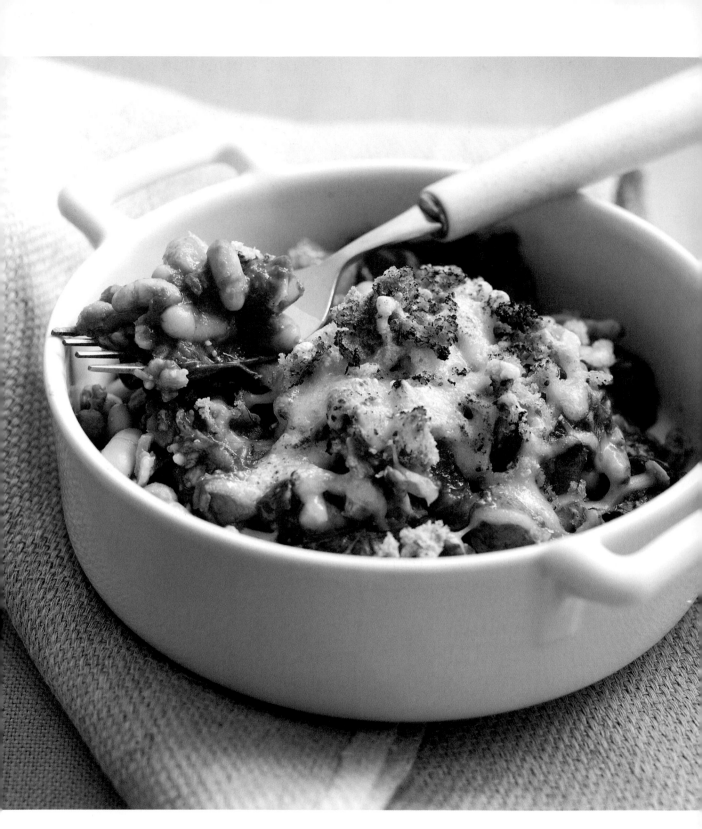

Chilli, Tomato, Oat and Bean Bake

A wholesome winter bake. For a variation add some vegetable stock to make a thick soup.

Serves 4–6

1 tablespoon olive oil
1 red onion, peeled and roughly chopped
2 garlic cloves, peeled and finely chopped
1 teaspoon fresh thyme leaves
1 teaspoon dried chilli flakes
800g tinned chopped tomatoes
400g tinned flageolet beans, drained and rinsed
125g whole, rolled porridge oats
2 handfuls (about 50g) baby spinach
125g frozen peas, defrosted
1 tablespoon reduced-salt soy sauce
freshly ground black pepper
50g Gruyère cheese, grated
4–6 tablespoons multi-seeded wholemeal
   breadcrumbs

1. Preheat the oven to 200°C/400°F/gas mark 6.

2. Heat the oil in a large non-stick saucepan, add the onion, garlic, thyme and chilli flakes and cook gently for 8–10 minutes until the onions have softened but not coloured.

3. Stir in the tomatoes with 1 tin water, bring to the boil then reduce to a simmer. Add the beans and oats and cook gently, stirring regularly, for about 5 minutes until slightly thickened.

4. Fold in the spinach and peas until the spinach has wilted. Add the soy sauce and season to taste with pepper.

5. Spoon the mixture into individual gratin dishes. Mix together the cheese and bread-crumbs in a bowl and sprinkle over the top. Bake for 10–15 minutes or until bubbling and golden.

Per portion: 371 kcal, 11g fat, 3.1g sat fat, 0.32g sodium, 54g carbohydrate

Roasted Peperonata with Cannellini Beans

This makes a delicious starter either warm or cold and also a good accompaniment to grilled meats. For a more substantial vegetarian supper, top it with a poached egg.

To roast peppers, cook them in a hot oven – 200°C/400°F/gas mark 6 for about 20 minutes – or char-grill them until well-blistered.

SERVES 6

2 tablespoons extra virgin olive oil
3 onions, peeled and sliced
4 garlic cloves, peeled and finely chopped
3 red peppers, roasted, deseeded, peeled
   and sliced
3 yellow peppers, roasted, deseeded, peeled
   and sliced
3 plum tomatoes, diced
410g tinned cannellini beans in water, drained
   and rinsed
4 anchovy fillets, rinsed and diced
1 hot red chilli, deseeded and finely diced
25g baby capers, rinsed
6 basil leaves, roughly torn
3 tablespoons freshly chopped flat-leaf parsley
1 tablespoon balsamic vinegar
freshly ground black pepper

1. Heat the oil in a large frying pan, add the onions and garlic and fry for about 10 minutes until the onions have softened but not coloured.

2. Add the peppers, tomatoes, beans, anchovies, chilli and capers and cook, uncovered, for a further 10 minutes.

3. Fold in the basil, parsley and balsamic vinegar. Season to taste.

Per portion: 155 kcal, 5g fat, 0.7g sat fat, 0.13g sodium, 23g carbohydrate

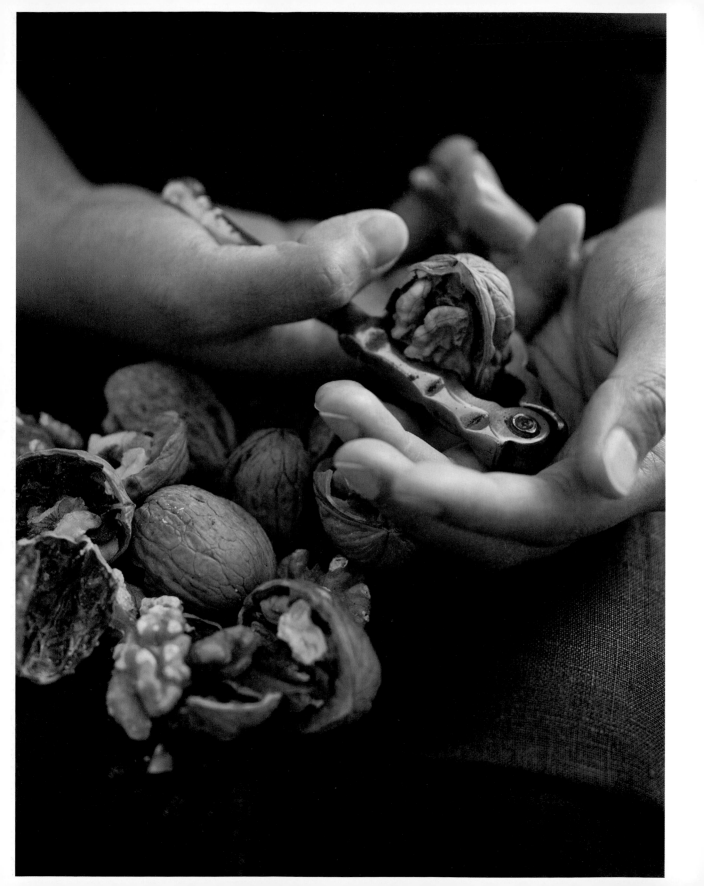

Nuts and seeds

About nuts and seeds

Nuts and seeds have a low GI and thanks to their low carbohydrate content they also have a low GL. Seeds are a valuable source of protein, iron, calcium and omega 3 fatty acids. From the botanical point of view, peanuts (groundnuts) are a legume (see page 50), as they grow underground, but they have many similarities to other nuts. Linseeds and hemp seeds are useful for the essential fatty acids they contain. These are good for the skin and brain and for the joints. Toasting nuts and seeds in the oven or in a dry frying pan will enhance their flavour.

Snacks

Nuts and seeds can make satisfying snacks, but because of their calorie content, you should not eat more than 25g as a portion. Rather than eat them by the handful, try eating them one by one!

Nut butters

Nut butters are useful as spreads to give added flavour and a sustained feeling of fullness. Because of their high calorie content you should limit your intake to a maximum of a tablespoon a day. You can buy both smooth and crunchy varieties of peanut butter as well as hazelnut and almond butter.

Tahini is not strictly a nut butter but a paste made from sesame seeds and is a good source of calcium.

Nut and seed oils

Oils are made from both nuts and seeds, and like all fats and oils, they contain no carbohydrate and thus have a GI and GL of 0 (see page 16). They are quite high in calories, with 100g providing almost 900 kcal, so you should only use them in small amounts. Nut oils such as walnut oil can be used to add flavour. Oil made from peanuts is often called groundnut oil.

Coconut oil is very high in saturated fat, rapeseed oil is a good source of monounsaturates and sesame, soya and sunflower seed oils all contain a higher proportion of polyunsaturates.

Storage

The fat in nuts and seeds makes them go rancid if you keep them too long, so make sure that any you buy have a long shelf life and store them in an airtight container in a cool, dry place.

Nuts and seeds in the recipes

If you cannot find the type of nut or seed specified in a recipe try another one, for example use sunflower seeds instead of pumpkin seeds. You can also add a different flavour by toasting the nuts and seeds, as in the recipe for Dukkah (see opposite). Try your own variations.

Calorie content

Nuts and seeds have a relatively high calorie (kcal) level due to the amount of oils they contain.

Almonds 612 kcal per 100g

Brazil nuts 682 kcal per 100g

Cashew nuts 611 kcal per 100g

Chestnuts 170 kcal per 100g

Coconut, desiccated 604 kcal per 100g

Hazelnuts 650 kcal per 100g

Macadamia nuts 748 kcal per 100g

Peanuts 563 kcal per 100g

Pecans 689 kcal per 100g

Pine nuts 688 kcal per 100g

Sesame seeds 618 kcal per 100g

Sunflower seeds 581 kcal per 100g

Chicken Satay Sticks

SERVES 4

450g skinless, boneless chicken breast fillets,
  cut into thin strips

MARINADE
1 lemongrass stalk, tender inner part only,
  finely chopped
2 shallots, peeled and chopped
2 garlic cloves, peeled and chopped
1cm piece fresh ginger, peeled and chopped
2 teaspoons raw cane soft brown sugar
1 teaspoon ground turmeric
½ teaspoon ground cumin
½ teaspoon ground coriander
1 tablespoon vegetable oil

SAUCE
150g crunchy peanut butter
2 tablespoon reduced-salt soy sauce
2 tablespoon clear honey
2 tablespoon rice vinegar
6 tablespoons freshly chopped coriander

1. For the marinade, put all the ingredients in a
food-processor with 2 tablespoons water and
whizz to a paste. Toss the chicken strips in the
marinade to coat each piece well. Cover and
leave in a cool place for at least 1 hour or up to
24 hours in the fridge. Remove from the fridge
1 hour before cooking.

2. For the sauce, mix all the ingredients together
and thin with a little water, if necessary.

3. When ready to cook the chicken, preheat the
grill to high. Thread the chicken strips onto
8 bamboo skewers and cook for 7–8 minutes,
turning once until cooked through. Serve with
the sauce and an oriental-style salad of
cucumber, beansprouts, radishes and carrot.

**Per portion: 273 kcal, 13g fat, 2.3g sat fat, 0.26g
sodium, 8g carbohydrate**

Dukkah

A wonderful mixture of nuts and seeds that can
be sprinkled on salads to enhance the flavour but
is traditionally served with chunks of bread lightly
dipped in oil then dunked in the dukkah. Great as
a snack but also a good accompaniment to a bowl
of soup for lunch or a light supper, or scattered
over vegetables and salads.

MAKES 200G (10–12 SERVINGS)

100g shelled hazelnuts in their skins
50g seeds – choose from sesame, sunflower,
  pumpkin (a mixture is fine)
25g coriander seeds
1 tablespoon cumin seeds

1. Place a medium-sized, dry frying pan over a
medium–high heat and add the hazelnuts. Stir
frequently until the skins begin to toast and fall
off and the nuts are lightly golden. Remove from
the pan.

2. Add the sesame, sunflower or pumpkin seeds
to the pan and toast until golden. stirring
frequently. Add to the hazelnuts.

3. Finally, put the coriander and cumin seeds in
the pan and toast lightly, stirring all the time.

4. Combine all the ingredients and pulse to a
very coarse powder in a food-processor or coffee
grinder. Allow to cool then store in an airtight
container. Will keep for up to 1 month.

**Per portion: 94 kcal, 10g fat, 0.8g sat fat, 0g sodium,
1g carbohydrate**

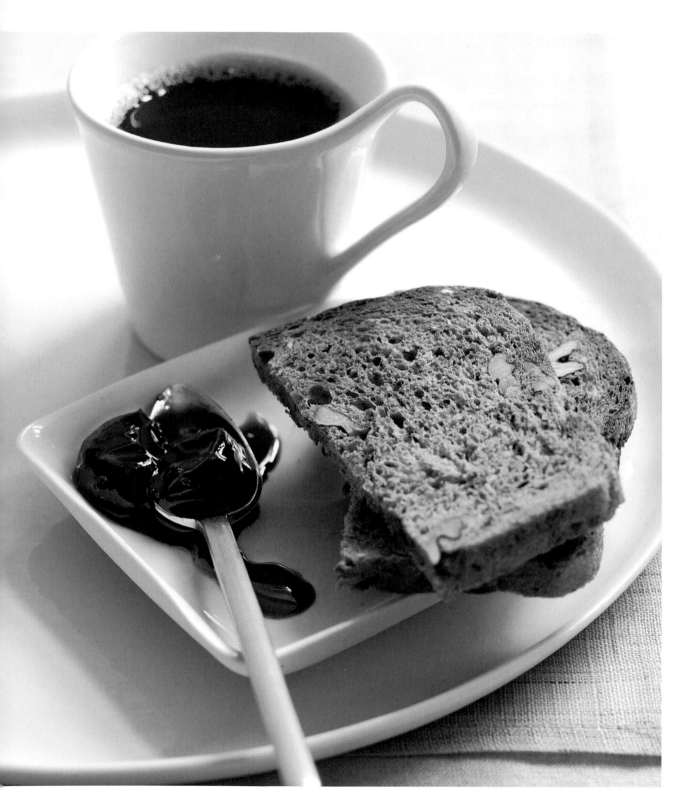

Walnut Bread

The salt helps the gluten to develop, which means the bread rises well. The walnut bread is shown opposite with Greek Cherry Glyko (page 149).

MAKES 2 LOAVES (20–24 slices each, including crust)

1kg strong brown bread flour with malted
    wheatgrains
1 sachet easy-blend dried yeast
2 teaspoons salt
600ml hand-hot water
100g walnut pieces

1. Put the flour, yeast and salt in a bowl and mix thoroughly. Make a well in the centre and add the water slowly, mixing to a soft dough. You may need to add 1–2 tablespoons more water. Knead for 10 minutes (5 with an electric mixer with a dough hook) on a lightly floured surface until smooth and elastic. Work in the walnuts.

2. Transfer to a lightly oiled polythene bag and leave in a warm place until doubled in size (you can omit this first proving if you're in a hurry!).

3. Halve the dough, knead each piece lightly again, then shape into oblongs and transfer to two lightly greased 900g loaf tins. Cover with polythene and leave to rise in a warm place until doubled in size – about 1 hour.

4. Meanwhile, preheat the oven to 220°C/425°F/ gas mark 7 and bake for 30–35 minutes until crusty and the bases sound hollow when tapped. Leave to cool on a wire rack then wrap in foil.

VARIATION – MULTISEED BREAD
Replace the walnuts with 2 tablespoons each of linseed, millet, sunflower seeds, poppy seeds, sesame seeds and pumpkin seeds.

Per slice without seeds: 98 kcal, 3g fat, 0.5g sat fat, 0.30g sodium, 15g carbohydrate
Per slice with seeds: 105 kcal, 3g fat, 0.7g sat fat, 0.30g sodium, 15g carbohydrate

Seeded Soda Bread Rolls

Quick and easy to make and perfect to go with soups and salads, these rolls also freeze well. If wished, use commercially prepared buttermilk instead of souring your own milk.

MAKES 18

450ml milk
1 tablespoon fresh lemon juice
300g strong brown bread flour with
    malted wheatgrain
300g strong white bread flour with kibbled grains
    of wheat and rye
50g assorted seeds such as linseed, sesame,
    hemp, sunflower
1½ teaspoons bicarbonate of soda
1 teaspoon salt

1. Preheat the oven to 230°C/450°F/gas mark 8. Sour the milk by mixing it with the lemon juice and leaving it to stand for 15 minutes to thicken.

2. Mix the dry ingredients together in a large bowl. Make a well in the centre and add most of the soured milk.

3. Working from the centre, combine the mixture with either your hand or a wooden spoon, adding more of the soured milk if necessary. The dough should be soft but not too sticky.

4. Spoon the mixture into 18 small mounds on lightly greased baking trays and bake for 15–20 minutes until risen and golden and the rolls sound hollow when tapped on the base.

5. Transfer to a wire rack and cover with a clean tea towel. Leave until cool enough to eat. When cold, they may be stored in an airtight container for 2–3 days.

Per roll: 144 kcal, 3g fat, 0.9g sat fat, 0.19g sodium, 25g carbohydrate

Spiced Nut Fingers

A rich nutty biscuit to serve with coffee or with a pudding such as fruit salad.

MAKES ABOUT 72

2 eggs
200g caster sugar
¼ teaspoon natural vanilla extract
½ teaspoon ground cinnamon
½ teaspoon ground allspice
60g ready-to-eat dried apricots, finely chopped
175g ground almonds
125g shelled hazelnuts, ground
½ teaspoon baking powder
50g flaked almonds

1. Preheat the oven to 130°C/275°F/gas mark 1. Line 2 baking trays with baking parchment or non-stick baking plastic.

2. Whisk the eggs, caster sugar and vanilla until pale and thick. Fold in the spices, apricots, ground nuts and baking powder. Spoon into a large piping bag fitted with a 1cm plain nozzle and pipe the mixture in 5cm fingers onto the parchment paper, leaving a little room for spreading. Dot the top of each 'finger' with flaked almonds, then bake for about 30 minutes until lightly golden.

3. Remove from the oven and cool on wire racks. Store in an airtight container.

Per finger: 45 kcal, 3g fat, 0.3g sat fat, 0.01g sodium, 4g carbohydrate

Seeded Oat Thins

These biscuits are wheat free and perfect for a light snack with low-fat soft cheese or jam - they are photographed here with curd cheese. Store in an airtight container.

MAKES ABOUT 70

275g medium oatmeal
25g potato flour
1 tablespoon poppy seeds
1 tablespoon sesame seeds
2 tablespoons sesame oil

1. Preheat the oven to 180°C/350°F/gas mark 4.

2. Put the dry ingredients in a bowl and mix well. Pour in 250ml boiling water and the oil and, when cool enough to handle, mix to a firm dough. (Note: For a really low-fat version omit the oil and use 300ml boiling water.)

3. Allow to cool until just cool enough to handle then roll out very thinly on a very lightly floured surface.

4. Stamp out 6cm rounds and place on non-stick baking trays. Re-roll the trimmings as necessary. You may need to add a few more drops of water if the dough becomes slightly dry.

5. Bake for 20–25 minutes until completely dried out. Cool on wire racks. Store in an airtight container.

Per thin: 21 kcal, 1g fat, 0.1g sat fat, 0g sodium, 3g carbohydrate

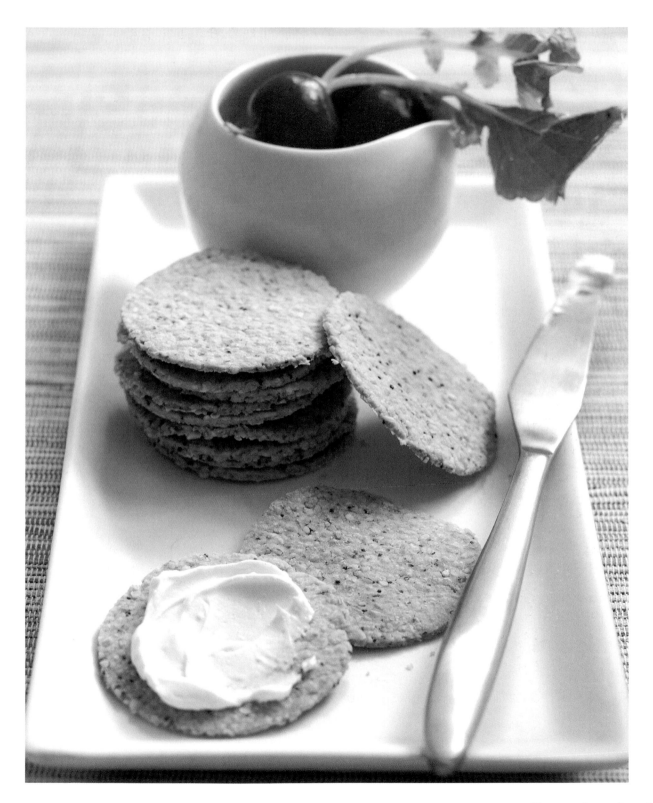

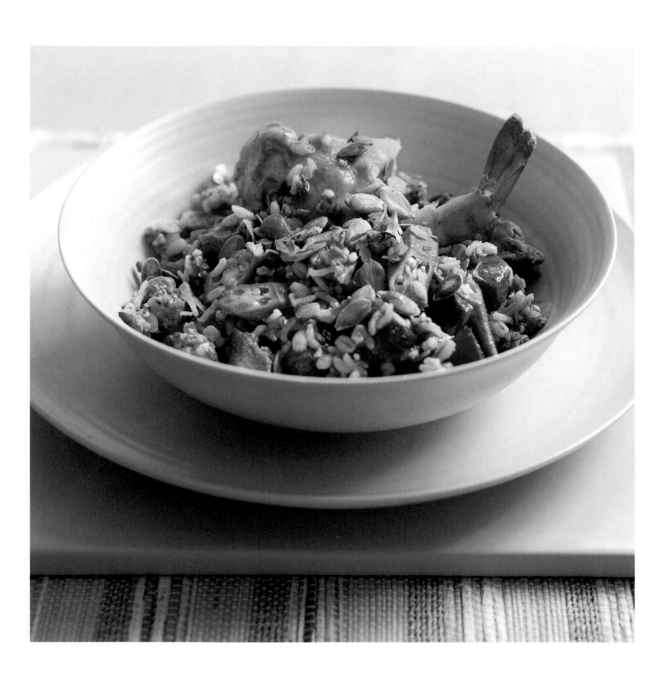

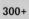

Mixed Grain Jambalaya

SERVES 4

4 skinless, boneless chicken thighs, halved
1 tablespoon seasoned potato flour
1 tablespoon vegetable oil
1 onion, peeled and finely chopped
1 garlic clove, peeled and finely chopped
½ red pepper, deseeded and chopped
½ green pepper, deseeded and chopped
1 teaspoon fresh thyme leaves
1 red chilli, deseeded and roughly chopped
50g wholegrain brown barley, soaked in
    boiling water, then drained
230g tinned chopped tomatoes
500ml chicken stock
100g raw garlic sausage, roughly chopped
    and lightly dry-fried
100g raw chorizo, roughly chopped and
    lightly dry-fried
75g brown basmati rice, rinsed
25g millet seeds, dry-fried until they 'pop'
4 king-size prawns, peeled and deveined
25g pumpkin seeds
125g okra, sliced
2 tablespoons chopped parsley
freshly ground black pepper

1. Dust the chicken in the flour. Heat the oil in a large non-stick frying pan, then remove and set aside. Add the next six ingredients to the pan and cook over a medium heat to soften the onion.

2. Add the barley, tomatoes and chicken stock and bring to the boil. Add the chicken and sausages, with any juices. Lower the heat and stir in the rice and millet. Cook, covered, for 20 minutes or until the rice is almost tender. Remove the lid and simmer for a further 10 minutes.

3. Fold in the prawns, pumpkin seeds and okra and cook for a further 5 minutes. Finally add the parsley and season to taste.

**Per portion: 492 kcal, 20g fat, 5.9g sat fat,
0.79g sodium, 43g carbohydrate**

Curried Prawns and Beans with Cashew Nuts

A very quick supper dish with loads of flavour. It is the perfect food when served with basmati rice.

SERVES 4

250g runner beans, strings removed and cut
    in thin slices
8 spring onions, cut in 3cm pieces
2 garlic cloves, peeled and thinly sliced
1 tablespoon vegetable oil
2 green chillies, deseeded and cut in slices
1 teaspoon mustard seeds
75g unsalted cashew nuts
½ teaspoon ground turmeric
½ teaspoon ground cumin
½ teaspoon ground coriander
400ml tinned reduced-fat coconut milk
400g raw peeled prawns
1 teaspoon garam masala
coriander leaves, to garnish
sliced red chillies, to garnish (optional)

1. Blanch the beans in boiling water for 5 minutes, drain and refresh under cold water. Drain again and set aside.

2. Fry the spring onions and garlic in the oil over a medium heat for 6 minutes. Add the chillies, mustard seeds and cashew nuts, increase the heat and cook for a further 5 minutes until the onions have turned pale golden.

3. Add the spices and coconut milk. Cook until the coconut milk has reduced by about one third. Add the blanched beans and the prawns and simmer, covered, for 3 minutes, until the prawns have just turned pink. Stir in the garam masala.

4. Serve at once with brown basmati rice. Garnish with coriander leaves and red chillies, if wished.

**Per portion: 254 kcal, 14g fat, 2.5g sat fat,
0.31g sodium, 12g carbohydrate**

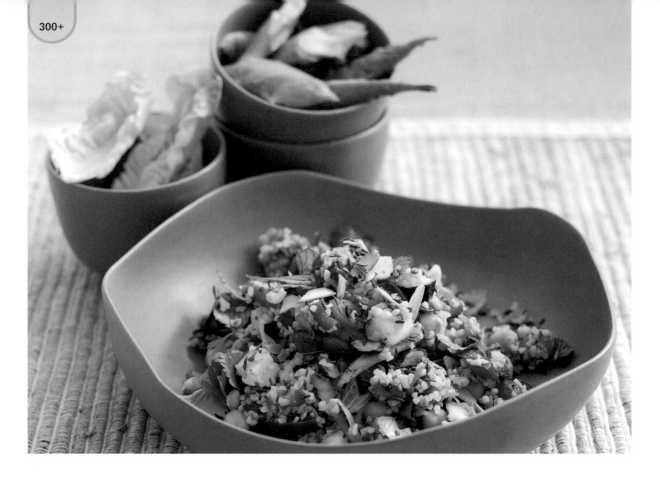

Spiced Tabbouleh with Smoked Mackerel

SERVES 4

1 tablespoon coriander seeds
1 tablespoon cumin seeds
2 roasted red peppers, diced
2 pickled chillies, thinly sliced
2 ripe tomatoes, diced
1 medium courgette, cut in 1cm dice
4 spring onions, thinly sliced
2 garlic cloves, peeled and finely chopped
400g tinned chick peas in water, drained and
   rinsed
1 tablespoon extra virgin olive oil
finely grated zest and juice of 2 limes
175g bulgur, rinsed, well drained, then left to soak
   in 200ml cold water
25g toasted flaked almonds

25g shelled pistachios, roughly chopped
handful of coriander leaves
16 mint leaves, shredded
100g smoked mackerel fillets, skinned and flaked

1. Dry-fry the seeds in a small frying pan until
fragrant, then crush and set aside. Combine the
peppers with the chillies, tomatoes, courgette,
onions, garlic and chick peas. Fold in the olive oil,
lime zest and juice. Season with pepper to taste.

2. Just before serving, add the vegetables with
their juices to the bulgur. Fold in the crushed
seeds, almonds, pistachios and herbs. Check the
seasoning and spoon into a large bowl. Scatter
with flakes of mackerel and serve with baby gem
lettuce leaves and lime wedges.

**Per portion: 461 kcal, 21g fat, 2.4g sat fat,
0.26g sodium, 52g carbohydrate**

A Green Stew with Roasted Walnuts

On a cold winter's night there's nothing better than a good stew, but stews don't need to contain meat; this one is thickened with porridge oats.

SERVES 4

1 tablespoon olive oil
1 onion, peeled, halved and thinly sliced
1 garlic clove, peeled and finely chopped
1 bulb of fennel, halved and thinly sliced
1 tablespoon fennel seeds
50g whole, rolled porridge oats
1 leek, thinly sliced
8 new potatoes, scrubbed, quartered lengthways
¼ Savoy cabbage, shredded
pinch of grated nutmeg
pinch of ground allspice
about 1 litre vegetable stock
50g frozen peas
75g small broccoli florets
50g walnut pieces, roasted at 180°C/350°F/gas mark 4 for 10–15 minutes.
freshly ground black pepper

1. Heat the olive oil in a large saucepan then add the onion, garlic, fennel and fennel seeds and cook over a medium heat for 7–8 minutes. Add the oats, increase the heat and cook, stirring regularly, until the oats have turned light golden.

2. Add the leek, potatoes, cabbage and spices and stir to combine. Cook for 3 minutes then add the stock. Bring to the boil, reduce the heat, cover and simmer for 15 minutes.

3. Add the peas and broccoli, return to the boil, stirring to combine, then simmer, covered, for 4 minutes or until the broccoli is just tender. Season to taste, sprinkle with walnuts and serve with chunks of seeded bread.

Per portion: 267 kcal, 14g fat, 1.4g sat fat, 0.32g sodium, 30g carbohydrate

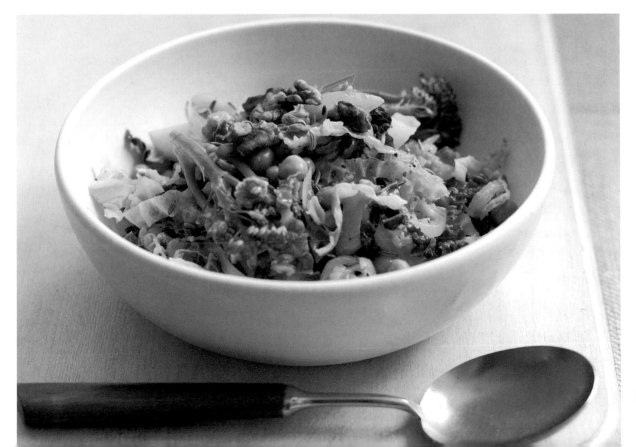

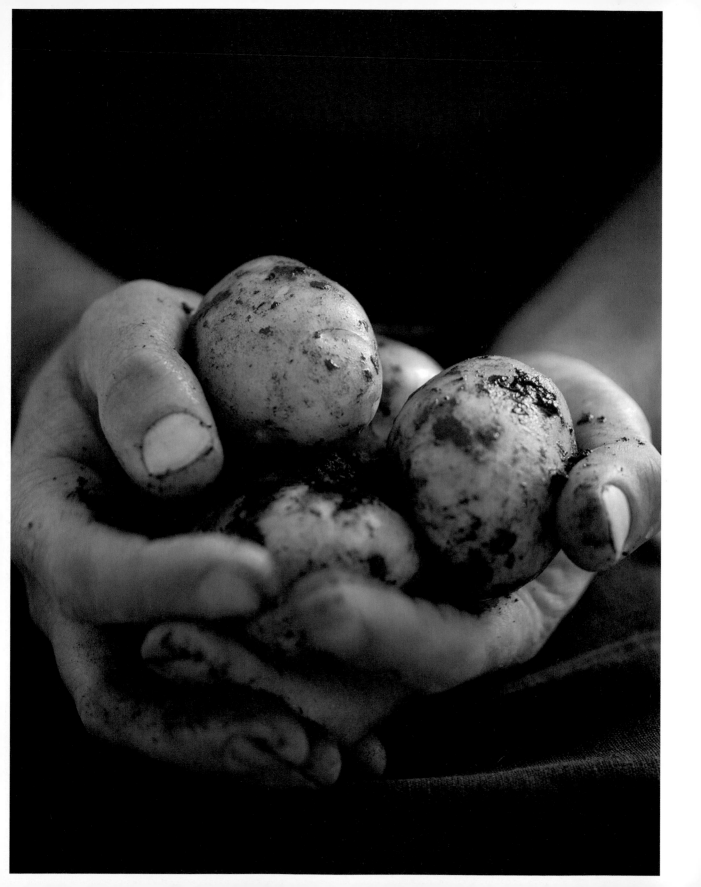

Vegetables

About vegetables

In the past we used to eat far more vegetables than we do today, especially potatoes and green vegetables. During the war years, even with the horrendous stresses of people's everyday lives, their diet was much healthier because they 'dug for victory' and ate lots of potatoes and home-grown vegetables.

Vegetables and 'five a day'

Vegetables are an important part of the 'five a day' fruit and vegetables that we are all encouraged to eat for good health. Potatoes are regarded nutritionally as a food that provides starchy carbohydrate than as part of the vegetable group, so they are not included in the five a day. All other vegetables are included though, even those with a high GL, so if you are following the low GL diet, you should try to combine them with low GL foods. For instance, try eating your mashed potatoes with a selection of brussels sprouts, baked onions and carrots, have a large side salad with your jacket potato and enjoy courgettes and parsnips together.

Where possible, just give vegetables a good scrub, instead of peeling, which retains many more nutrients, especially fibre. Locally and home-grown organic vegetables are a good choice.

Portion sizes for vegetables are approximately 3 tablespoons or 80g.

Potatoes

These are a good source of carbohydrate and are also relatively low in calories. But because they contain carbohydrate, they absorb fat easily so if they are fried or roasted in oil, their calorie content increases. The skin on potatoes is a good source of dietary fibre so it is best to cook them with their skins wherever possible. You can easily make roast potatoes and oven chips from potatoes with their skins; brush or spray them with a tiny amount of oil and bake in a hot oven.

Jacket potatoes are filling and economical and although they have a high GI, their GL is not so high. Try eating them with low GI fillings such as baked beans, chilli or other bean-based mixtures.

Small new potatoes cooked in their skins have a lower GI and GL so they are a good choice, while sweet potatoes have an even lower GI and GL. They have the added benefit of containing the antioxidant beta-carotene. Try them oven baked. If you do not like them, ordinary potatoes are an acceptable substitute.

Green and salad vegetables

All of the cabbages, broccoli, sprouts, lettuce, cucumber, tomatoes, radishes and cauliflower contain powerful antioxidants. They are low in carbohydrate and therefore have a negligible effect on your blood sugar levels, so eat large portions of them!

Frozen vegetables

When vegetables are frozen they retain all of those important vitamins so fill the freezer with peas, broad beans, sweetcorn and spinach and you will always have some ready to hand. If you have a glut of vegetables in the garden you can freeze your own after blanching them first.

Butternut Squash Curry with Coconut Milk

Reduced-fat coconut milk does not have the same thickening qualities as full-fat coconut milk so I have used ground peanuts to thicken the sauce at the end of the cooking time. Using four dried chillies gives a hot curry, but you can reduce the quantity if you want a milder version!

SERVES 4

2–4 dried hot red chillies, seeds discarded
6 spring onions, roughly chopped
2 large garlic cloves, peeled and chopped
2 stalks lemongrass, tender inner part only,
 finely chopped
1 tablespoon vegetable oil
2 teaspoons ground coriander
½ teaspoon ground turmeric
1 teaspoon paprika
400ml tinned reduced-fat coconut milk
150ml vegetable stock
1 medium butternut squash (about 750g) peeled,
 deseeded and cut in 5cm chunks
1 red pepper, halved, deseeded and
 cut in rough dice
2 green cardamom pods, crushed
1 cinnamon stick
1½ tablespoons reduced-salt soy sauce
1½ teaspoons raw cane brown sugar
1½ teaspoons lemon juice
25g raw peanuts, ground

1. Tear the chillies into small pieces and pour over enough boiling water from the kettle to cover. Set aside for 10 minutes to soften, then drain and place in a food-processor or liquidiser. Add the spring onions, garlic and lemongrass and blend to a paste, adding a little water as necessary.

2. Heat the oil in a large saucepan over a medium-low heat. Add the chilli mixture and cook, stirring, for about 5 minutes. Add the ground spices and cook for a further 1 minute. Stir in the coconut milk and simmer for 5 minutes, stirring frequently.

3. Stir in the stock and bring to a simmer. Add the squash, red pepper, cardamom and cinnamon. Simmer, partially covered, for 20–25 minutes until the squash is tender.

4. Stir in the remaining ingredients and simmer for 2–3 minutes. Serve with brown basmati rice.

Per portion: 255 kcal, 15g fat, 0.9g sat fat, 0.36g sodium, 26g carbohydrate

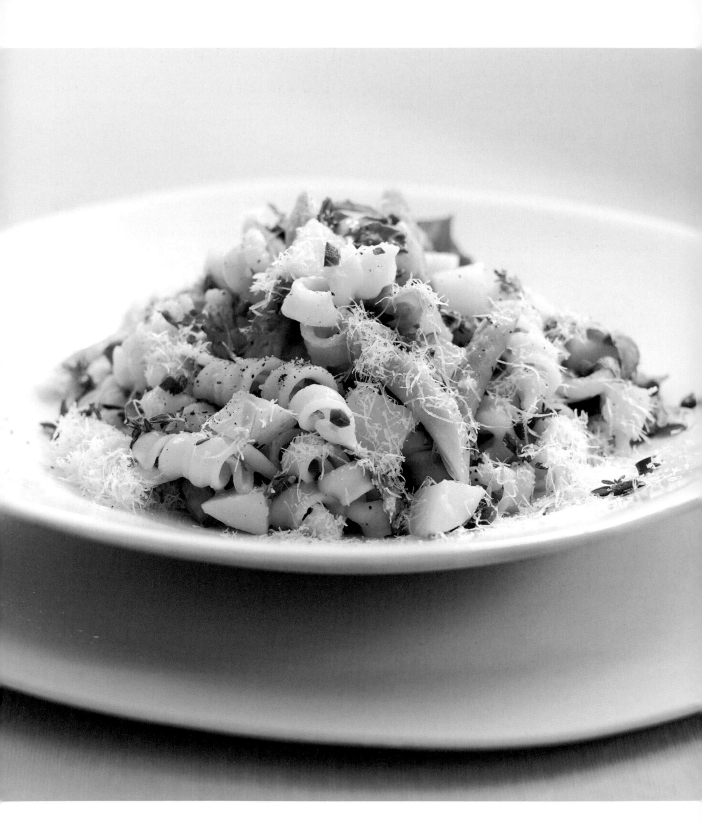

One-Pot Pasta with Potato, Green Beans and Rocket

One of my favourite comfort suppers, this recipe can be whipped up quickly if you have the ingredients in your storecupboard.

SERVES 4

1 tablespoon olive oil
1 onion, peeled and chopped
2 garlic cloves, peeled and chopped
250g potatoes, cut in small dice
100g green beans, cut in short lengths
1 tablespoon fresh thyme leaves
2 red chillies, deseeded and finely chopped
1 litre vegetable stock
250g dried pasta shapes
50g rocket, roughly chopped
50g freshly grated Parmesan
4 tablespoons freshly chopped basil leaves
freshly ground black pepper

1. Heat the oil in a very large saucepan, add the onion and cook for 2–3 minutes until softened. Add the garlic, potatoes, beans, thyme and chilli and cook, stirring, for 3–4 minutes, adding a little of the measured stock if the mixture starts to stick.

2. Pour in the stock and add the pasta. Bring to the boil and stir well. Simmer, partially covered for about 10 minutes until the potatoes and pasta are tender and most of the stock has been absorbed.

3. Stir in the rocket, Parmesan and basil and season to taste with pepper.

Per portion: 371 kcal, 8g fat, 3.0g sat fat, 0.40g sodium, 63g carbohydrate

Minestrone Verde

Another winter warmer, this is my low-GL version of the popular Italian vegetable soup. This tastes even better the next day!

SERVES 6

1 tablespoon vegetable oil
2 leeks, cut in thin slices and washed
2 sticks celery, sliced
2 garlic cloves, peeled and crushed
400g tinned chopped tomatoes
1.75 litres vegetable stock
75g dried macaroni
175g mixed green vegetables, such as peas,
    green beans and sugar snap peas, cut in
    3cm lengths
400g tinned flageolet beans, drained and rinsed
1 tablespoon pesto
freshly ground black pepper
6 tablespoons freshly grated Parmesan, to serve

1. Heat the oil in a large heavy-based saucepan. Add the leeks, celery and garlic and cook over a low heat for 6–8 minutes.

2. Add the tomatoes, stock and macaroni and bring to the boil, then cook, partially covered, for 8 minutes.

3. Stir in the green vegetables, flageolet beans and pesto and continue to cook for 2–3 minutes. Season with pepper and serve with grated Parmesan.

Per portion: 161 kcal, 5g fat, 0.8g sat fat, 0.48g sodium, 21g carbohydrate

Greek-Style Village Salad

Marinating the onions releases some of their juices to make a delicious dressing. Normally the Greeks use feta cheese in this salad, but it has a high sodium content so cottage cheese is a good alternative.

SERVES 4

1 red onion, peeled, halved lengthways and
    very thinly sliced
1 garlic clove, peeled and crushed
1 teaspoon dried oregano
1 teaspoon capers, chopped
1 tablespoon red wine vinegar
4 plum tomatoes, cut in chunks
½ cucumber, cut in quarters lengthways then
    roughly chopped
25g kalamata olives
125g cottage cheese
2 teaspoons fresh oregano leaves (optional)
freshly ground black pepper

1. Combine the onion, garlic, dried oregano, capers and vinegar and leave to marinate for at least 1 hour.

2. Put the tomatoes, cucumber and olives in a salad bowl and add the onion mixture. Add the cottage cheese, fresh oregano and plenty of pepper.

3. Fold through and serve at once – this is a salad that does not keep!

Per portion: 68 kcal, 2g fat, 0.5g sat fat, 0.25g sodium, 8g carbohydrate

Chunky Beetroot Soup with Kidney Beans

Keeping the vegetables chunky and leaving their skins on where possible as well as adding kidney beans makes this a nutritious and substantial soup. The addition of vinegar at the last minute brings back some of the characteristic pink colour to the beetroot. Serve with crusty bread.

SERVES 6–8

2 onions, peeled and roughly chopped
1 large carrot, chopped
1 large turnip, chopped
1 large parsnip, chopped
2 sticks celery, chopped
500g raw beetroot, peeled and chopped
3 garlic cloves, peeled and crushed
1 teaspoon fresh thyme leaves
1 low-salt vegetable stock cube
400g potatoes, diced
200g Savoy cabbage, shredded
410g tinned kidney beans in water, drained
    and rinsed
1 teaspoon freshly ground black pepper
1 tablespoon raspberry vinegar or red wine
    vinegar
150g 0% fat Greek yogurt, or low-fat
    fromage frais, to serve
freshly choppped dill, to garnish

1. Place the first nine ingredients in a large stockpot with 2 litres water. Bring to the boil then cover and simmer for 30 minutes.

2. Add the potatoes, cabbage, beans and pepper and simmer, covered, for a further 20–30 minutes until the potatoes are tender. Stir in the vinegar.

3. Serve in large bowls with a dollop of yogurt and a sprinkling of dill.

Per portion: 189 kcal, 1g fat, 0.1g sat fat, 0.43g sodium, 36g carbohydrate

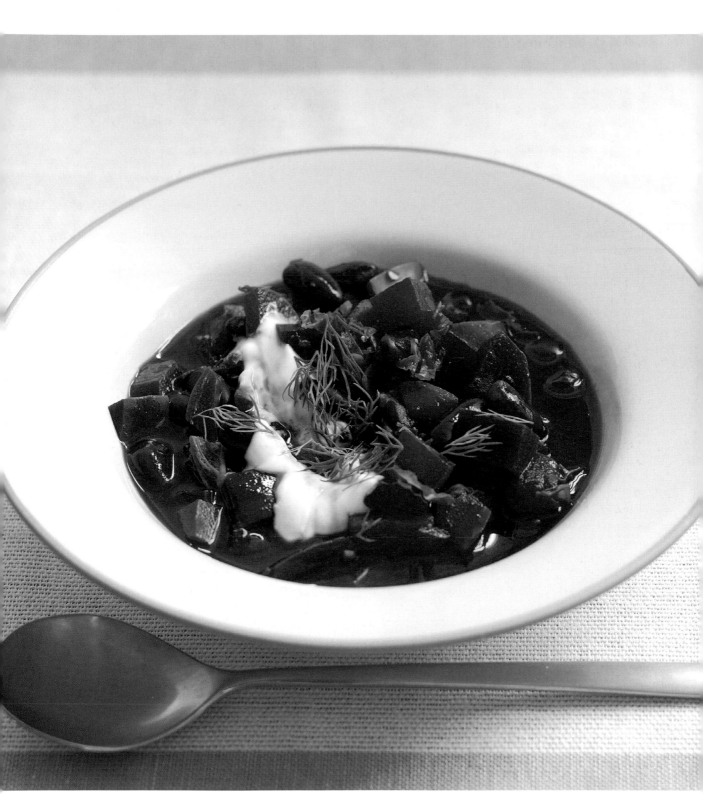

Vegetable Stir-Fry

A classic quick-and-easy recipe, this is a brilliant way to achieve your daily veg quota.

SERVES 2

1 tablespoon Hoisin sauce
1 tablespoon reduced-salt soy sauce
1 tablespoon hot chilli sauce
1 tablespoon sesame oil
1 large carrot, cut in ribbons
1 red pepper, cored and cut in 3cm pieces
125g button mushrooms
1 onion, peeled and chopped
250g mixed green vegetables, such as small
    broccoli florets, sugar snap peas, mangetout,
    very thinly sliced leeks, baby spinach
2 teaspoons cornflour mixed to a paste
    with 3 tablespoons water
juice of ½ lime
1 tablespoon sesame seeds

1. Mix the first three ingredients with
3 tablespoons water and set aside.

2. Heat the oil in a wok and add the carrot,
pepper, mushrooms and onion. Stir-fry over a
medium heat for 5 minutes. Add the green
vegetables and cook, stirring, for 2 minutes.

3. Add the reserved oriental mixture and cook
for 2 minutes.

4. Add the cornflour mixture and cook,
stirring for 1 minute.

5. Stir in the lime juice and sprinkle with the
sesame seeds. Serve at once with rice or noodles.

Per portion: 255 kcal, 10g fat, 1.5g sat fat,
0.42g sodium, 34g carbohydrate

Baby Roast Potatoes in Their Skins

Invest in a sheet of that wonderful non-stick,
heat-resistant baking 'plastic'. It will revolutionise
your baking – and is especially good for making
this recipe!

SERVES 4–6 as an accompaniment

1kg baby new potatoes in their skins, washed
1 tablespoon olive oil
½ head garlic, broken into cloves (optional)
a few sprigs of fresh thyme or rosemary
freshly ground black pepper
lemon juice (optional)

1. Preheat the oven to 200°C/400°F/gas mark 6.
Put the potatoes in a pan of cold water and bring
to the boil. Drain well.

2. Line a medium roasting tin with a sheet of
non-stick baking plastic (see above). Add the
potatoes and toss with the oil, garlic, herbs and
pepper to taste.

3. Roast in the oven for about 30 minutes,
shaking occasionally, until tender. Serve
sprinkled with a little lemon juice, if wished

Per portion: 203 kcal, 4g fat, 0.7g sat fat, 0.03g sodium,
41g carbohydrate

Bashed Carrots with Assorted Seeds and Lemon

The savoury seeds spice up this everyday vegetable and complement the sweet, tender carrots. Toasting seeds really brings out their flavour.

SERVES 4 as an accompaniment

500g carrots, roughly chopped
1 tablespoon hemp seeds
1 teaspoon caraway seeds
1 tablespoon lemon juice
freshly ground black pepper

1. Steam or cook the carrots in boiling water until just tender – about 15 minutes.

2. Meanwhile, put the seeds in a small non-stick frying pan over a medium heat and cook until lightly toasted and fragrant.

3. Drain the carrots thoroughly and return to the pan. Using a potato masher, roughly mash the carrots then stir in the remaining ingredients.

Per portion: 60 kcal, 2g fat, 0.1g sat fat, 0.03g sodium, 10g carbohydrate

Sweet Potato Mash with Dijon Mustard and Spring Onions

You can also make this recipe using traditional potatoes cooked in their skins. Either way they're delicious with sausages! For a perfectly balanced meal serve each portion with two grilled sausages, a wedge of braised cabbage (page 85) and a piece of fruit to finish.

SERVES 6 as an accompaniment

1.5kg sweet potatoes
1 bunch spring onions, chopped
150ml semi-skimmed milk
3 tablespoons Dijon mustard

1. Peel and cut the potatoes into even-sized chunks. Steam or cook in boiling water until tender – 15–20 minutes.

2. Put the spring onions and milk in a small saucepan and simmer very gently, covered, for about 5 minutes.

3. Drain and return the potatoes to the pan to dry out over a low heat. Roughly mash, then stir in the onions with their liquid and the mustard.

Per portion: 241 kcal, 2g fat, 0.6g sat fat, 0.23g sodium, 55g carbohydrate

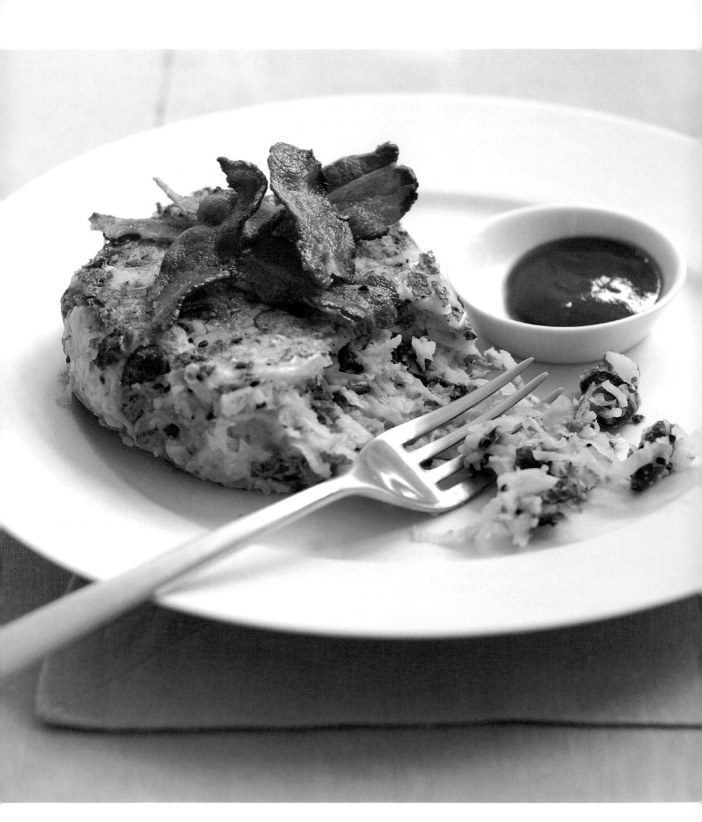

Bubble and Squeak Bean Cakes

Great as a brunch dish with (dare I say?) brown sauce or tomato ketchup! Black onion seeds are traditionally used in Indian cooking and are available in supermarkets and in Asian stores. A little crispy pancetta makes a great addition.

SERVES 4

250g large new potatoes, roughly chopped
250g Savoy cabbage or curly kale, shredded
1 small leek (about 100g) shredded
410g tinned kidney beans in water, drained and rinsed
2 teaspoons black onion seeds (kalonji)
freshly ground black pepper
4 teaspoons olive oil

1. Steam or cook the potatoes in boiling water until tender – about 15 minutes. Drain thoroughly and transfer to a large bowl. Reserve the cooking water and use to cook the cabbage and leeks for 5 minutes. Drain thoroughly.

2. Mash the potatoes and beans together then add the cabbage and leeks, onion seeds and plenty of pepper. Mix together and form into 4 large cakes.

3. Heat the oil in a large non-stick frying pan and fry the 'cakes' over a medium heat for about 5 minutes, turning once, until crisp and golden on both sides. Serve at once.

Per portion: 153 kcal, 4g fat, 0.6g sat fat, 0.25g sodium, 24g carbohydrate

Braised Red Cabbage

Traditionally, red cabbage is braised until it is very tender. This version is slightly crisper and is delicious served with low-fat sausages, pork, poultry and game.

SERVES 6–8 as an accompaniment

1 medium red cabbage (about 750g)
1 onion, peeled and chopped
15g unsalted butter
300ml vegetable stock
50ml red wine vinegar
1 tablespoon redcurrant jelly
2 tablespoons raw cane brown sugar
2 medium cooking apples, quartered, cored and chopped

1. Preheat the oven to 180°C/350°F/gas mark 4.

2. Shred the cabbage and place in a casserole dish with the onion, butter, stock and vinegar. Mix well then cover and cook in the oven for 1 hour.

3. Stir in the redcurrant jelly, sugar and apples and cook for a further 30 minutes.

Per portion: 101 kcal, 3g fat, 1.3g sat fat, 0.23g sodium, 19g carbohydrate

Spanish-Style Spinach with Walnuts and Cumin

Spinach provides a great variety of vitamins and minerals and is so easy to incorporate into dishes.

SERVES 4 as an accompaniment

750g spinach, washed and well drained
1 tablespoon olive oil
3 garlic cloves, peeled and thinly sliced
50g walnut pieces or pine nuts
2 teaspoons cumin seeds
½ teaspoon paprika
large pinch of saffron threads
75g seeded bread, toasted and torn in small
   pieces
1 tablespoon sherry vinegar
freshly ground black pepper

1. Tear large spinach leaves as necessary. Put a large pan over a medium heat and add the spinach, a handful at a time, stirring until wilted. Drain thoroughly and keep warm.

2. Heat the oil in a non-stick frying pan and add the garlic, walnuts, cumin seeds, paprika and saffron threads. Cook over a medium heat until the garlic is lightly golden, then stir in the pieces of bread.

3. Season the spinach to taste with vinegar and black pepper then sprinkle with the bread and nut mixture. Serve at once.

Per portion: 211 kcal, 14g fat, 1.4g sat fat, 0.37g sodium, 13g carbohydrate

Leek Stew

Long, slow cooking is required for chunks of leek in much the same way as for meat. The leeks should be unctuous by the end of it!

SERVES 4

1 tablespoon oil
1kg leeks, cut in 3cm chunks and washed
1 onion, peeled and chopped
2 garlic cloves, peeled and chopped
½ teaspoon cayenne pepper
25g black olives, pitted and chopped
400g tinned chopped tomatoes
410g tinned borlotti beans in water, drained
   and rinsed
1 ball light mozzarella, diced
12 large basil leaves, torn into small pieces

1. Preheat the oven to 180°C/350°F/gas mark 4. Heat the oil in a large flameproof casserole and add the leeks, onion, garlic and cayenne. Cover and cook over a medium heat for 10 minutes, adding a dash of water if necessary to prevent sticking.

2. Add the olives and tomatoes plus ½ tin of water and the beans. Bring to a simmer. Cover, transfer to the oven and cook for about 1 hour until the leeks are tender.
   If preferred, simmer gently on top of the stove for 1–1½ hours.

3. Stir in the mozzarella and basil. Serve with brown rice.

Per portion: 231 kcal, 8g fat, 0.7g sat fat, 0.21g sodium, 24g carbohydrate

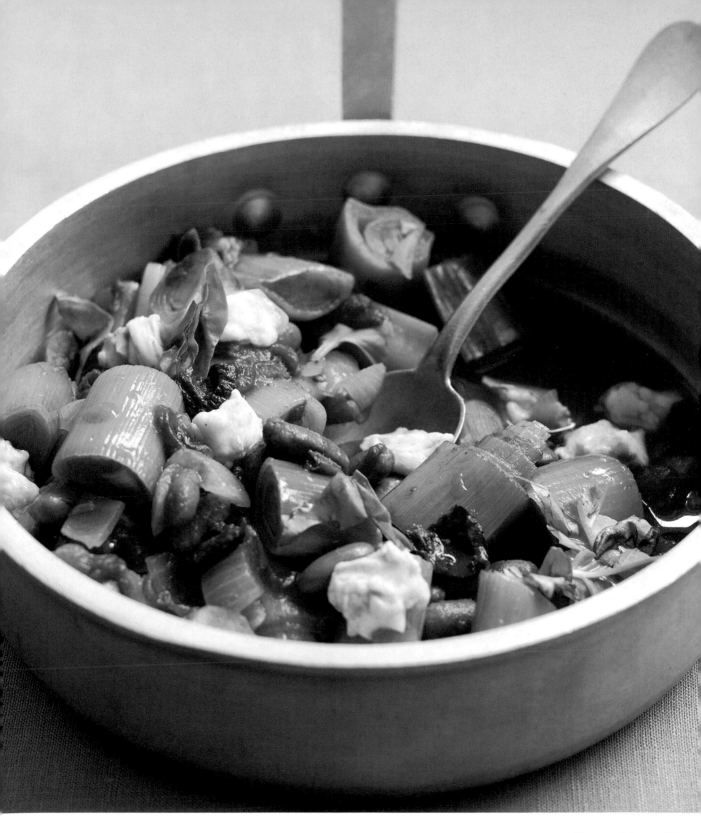

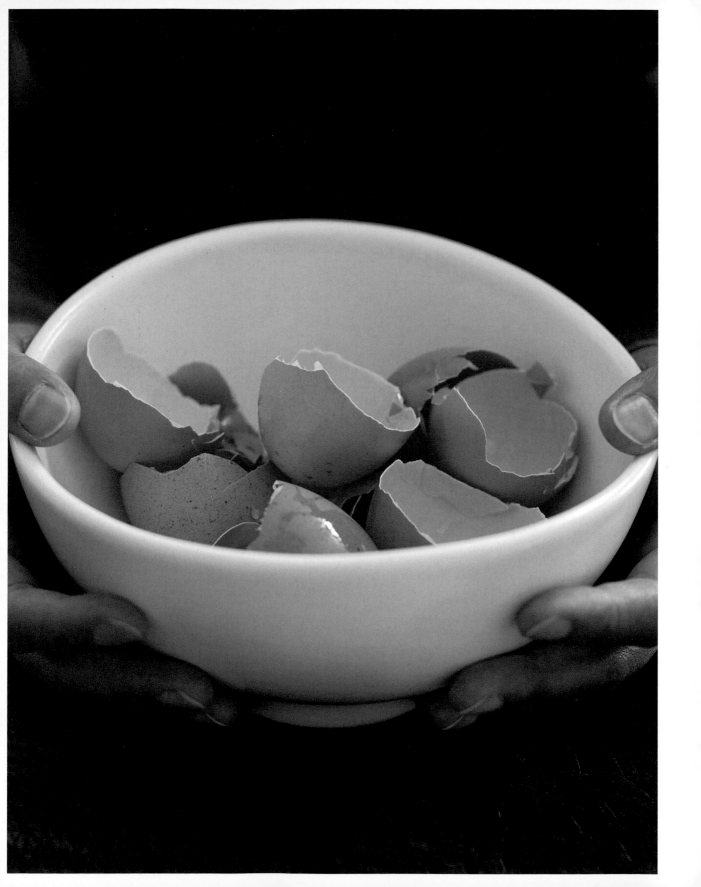

Eggs and dairy

About eggs and dairy

Eggs

Eggs are a pure protein food and thus have a GI of 0, and because they also contain no carbohydrate, they have a GL of 0. They are a useful basis for meals as well as a vital ingredient in cakes and puddings.

They do contain fat and cholesterol but this is found in the egg yolk so you can have a greater quantity of egg white. If you have an egg intolerance, use egg replacers.

Milk

Milk contains small quantities of the sugar lactose and is a good source of calcium in the diet. It has both a low GI and a low GL.

Full-cream milk is higher in calories than semi-skimmed or skimmed milk so is best avoided.

If you have an intolerance to cow's milk, use soya milk or other cow's milk substitutes in the recipes instead. Choose the varieties with added calcium.

Children and milk

Always give young children under 2 years of age full-cream milk to drink. Fully skimmed milk can be introduced at 5 years. Ask your health professional for advice.

Cream

Cream is best avoided, as it is particularly high in calories.

Yogurt and soya desserts

The majority of yogurts are made from cow's milk but Greek yogurt is traditionally made from ewe's milk. To save calories choose a plain low-fat yogurt and add your own fresh fruit or a home-made fruit jam such as the Greek Cherry Glyko (page 149).

Other dairy foods

Ice creams, custards, blancmanges, fromage frais, tofu, quark and other milk-based puddings all make tasty desserts.

Once again, to save calories, choose low-fat varieties and use semi-skimmed milk to make rice puddings and custards.

Cheese

All cheeses are a good source of calcium and protein and have a GI and GL of 0 as they do not contain carbohydrate. Cream cheese is particularly high in calories and hard cheeses are also quite high. Good-quality, well-matured hard cheeses are an excellent choice for adding flavour as you do not have to use a lot. Cottage cheese is low in calories so can be used more freely. Always check the labels as the calorie content can vary considerably between cheeses.

Dairy products per 100g

FOOD	CALORIES (kcal)	GI	CARBOHY-DRATES (g)	GL
Camembert	290	0	0	0
Cheddar	416	0	0	0
Cheddar, half fat	273	0	0	0
Cottage cheese	101	0	2	0
Cream cheese	439	0	0	0
Edam	341	0	0	0
Edam, half fat	229	0	0	0
Feta	250	0	0	0
Mozzarella	257	0	0	0
Parmesan	415	0	0	0
Stilton	410	0	0	0
Butter	744	0	0	0
Custard, skimmed milk	104	35	16	6
Custard, whole milk	118	35	16	6
Cream, double	496	0	2	0
Yogurt, low fat with sugar	78	31	8	2
Yogurt, low fat no sugar	47	14	7	1
Ice cream, full fat	177	61	17	10
Soya yogurt	72	50	13	7
Milk, skimmed	32	32	4	1
Milk, semi-skimmed	46	32	5	2
Milk whole	66	31	5	2

Spinach Raita

A delicious dip to serve with mini poppadoms, corn chips or crudités.

SERVES 4

1 x 225g bag baby spinach, washed and drained
1 teaspoon cumin seeds
1 tablespoon pine nuts
300g 0% Greek yogurt
1 garlic clove, peeled and crushed
4 large dates, finely chopped
4 large ready-to-eat dried apricots, finely chopped
½ teaspoon cayenne pepper

1. Put the spinach in a large saucepan over a high heat and stir until just wilted. Allow to cool then squeeze out the excess liquid and chop the spinach.

2. Put the cumin seeds and pine nuts in a small frying pan and toast over a medium heat, stirring frequently.

3. Combine the spinach, seeds and nuts with the remaining ingredients, mix well and serve.

Per portion: 109 kcal, 2g fat, 0.1g sat fat, 0.01g sodium, 15g carbohydrate

Piperade

A great brunch dish, this can be prepared to the end of step 2 then reheated and finished as required. Seeded soda bread rolls (page 67) make a good accompaniment.

SERVES 4

1 tablespoon olive oil
350g onion, peeled and thinly sliced
1 garlic clove, peeled and finely chopped
1 teaspoon thyme leaves
1 red pepper, deseeded and cut into thin strips
1 green pepper, deseeded and cut into thin strips
6 tomatoes, chopped
6 eggs, beaten
freshly ground black pepper
8 thin slices Bayonne or Parma ham (optional)

1. Heat the oil in a large non-stick frying pan and cook the onion, garlic and thyme until softened – about 10 minutes. You may need to add a few tablespoons of water to stop the ingredients sticking. Add the peppers and cook for a further 10 minutes, then add the tomatoes.

2. Cover the pan and cook for a further 10 minutes, until all the ingredients are soft and well combined.

3. When ready to eat, pour in the eggs and cook, stirring, over a medium heat until the eggs are lightly scrambled. Season to taste with pepper and serve hot with slices of ham on the side, if wished.

Per portion: 227 kcal, 13g fat, 3.3g sat fat, 0.14g sodium, 15g carbohydrate

Cheese and Pear Wraps

These are great for a lunchbox or picnic, but if you happen to be at home then wrap them in foil and heat through in a hot oven for 5 minutes, or in cling film for 1 minute on a high setting in the microwave.

SERVES 2

2 x 23cm soft tortillas
1 ball light mozzarella, diced
25g Parmesan. freshly grated
1 medium pear, cored and diced
4 sun-dried tomatoes, finely chopped
25g roasted chopped hazelnuts
watercress sprigs, to serve

1. Lay the tortillas on a flat surface. Combine all the remaining ingredients except the watercress in a bowl then divide between the tortillas, making a pile in the centre of each and leaving the edges free.

2. Roll up the tortillas tightly, folding in the sides as you go. Wrap in cling film or foil and keep in a cool place until required.

3. Cut in half and serve with watercress sprigs.

Per portion: 463 kcal, 26g fat, 4.1g sat fat, 0.38g sodium, 37g carbohydrate

Poached Eggs with Ham, Tomato and Watercress

A great brunch dish. Try adding ½ teaspoon of vinegar to the water when poaching the eggs – it helps to keep the whites firm.

SERVES 2

2 very fresh eggs
2 slices bread from a large seeded loaf
2 plum tomatoes at room temperature,
    thickly sliced
40g watercress
2 thin slices cooked ham (smoked if preferred)
freshly ground black pepper

1. Half-fill a wide saucepan with boiling water and add a dash of vinegar, if wished (see above). Place over a low heat so the water is kept at a simmer.

2. Break each egg into a small cup or ramekin. Stir the water in the saucepan gently to make a small 'whirlpool' then allow that to almost subside before carefully sliding the egg into the centre. Simmer for 2 minutes. Repeat to poach the second egg. Drain on kitchen paper, if you like.

3. Meanwhile, toast the bread and set a slice on each plate. Top with the tomato, watercress and ham. Carefully transfer an egg to the top of each and season generously with pepper. Serve at once.

Per portion: 225 kcal, 10g fat, 2.6g sat fat, 0.64g sodium, 18g carbohydrate

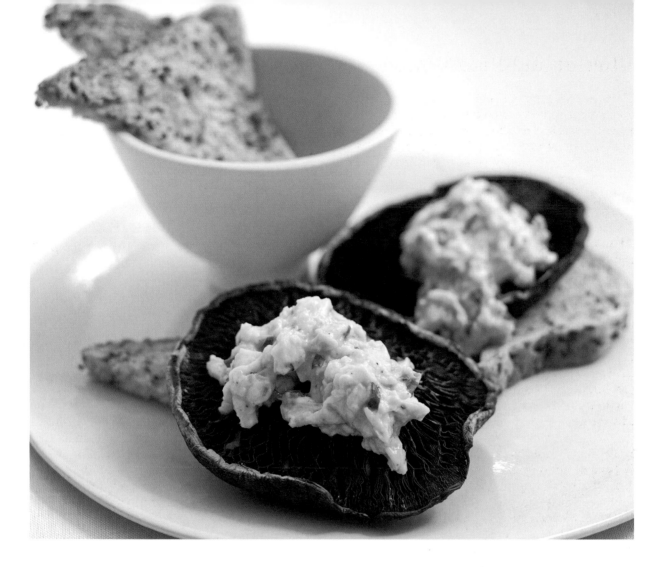

Scrambled Eggs on Grilled Field Mushrooms

A classic breakfast idea. Tarragon goes extremely well with eggs. Serve with seeded rolls (page 67) or toast.

SERVES 1

2 large field mushrooms (75–100g each), wiped
½ teaspoon vegetable oil
½ teaspoon unsalted butter
2 eggs
1 tablespoon freshly chopped herbs, such as
    basil, tarragon or chives
freshly ground black pepper

1. Preheat the grill to high. Brush the mushrooms with oil and season with pepper. Grill for about 10 minutes, turning once, until tender.

2. Meanwhile, melt the butter in a small non-stick pan. Whisk the eggs with a fork and season with pepper. Add to the pan and cook, stirring, over a gentle heat until lightly scrambled. Stir in the herbs and serve at once piled onto the mushrooms.

Per portion: 224 kcal, 17g fat, 5.2g sat fat, 0.17g sodium, 1g carbohydrate

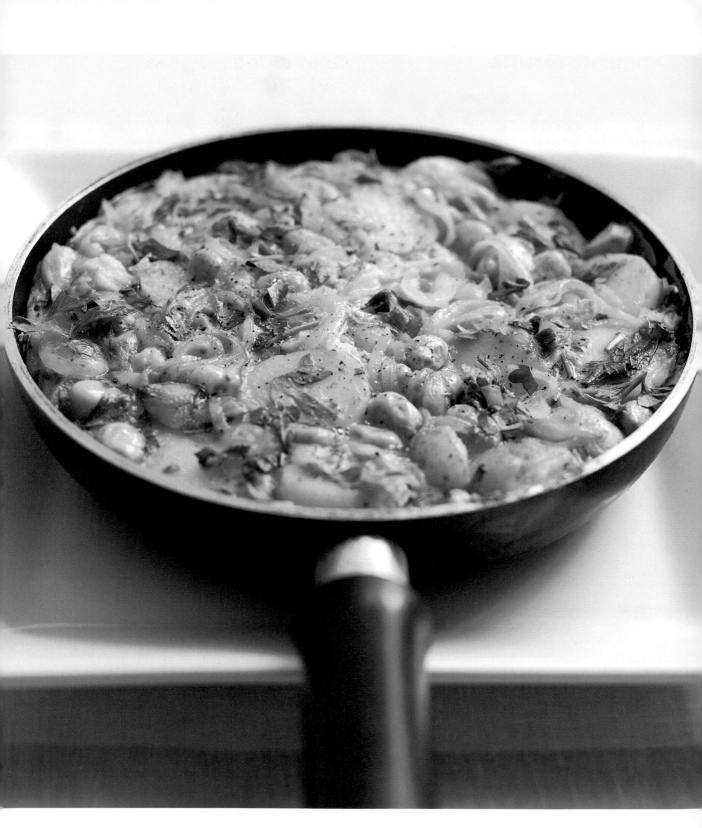

Spanish Tortilla

This is a variation of the classic onion and potato flavouring. In Spain, Tortilla is served in small squares as a tapas with drinks or between two chunky slices of fresh bread. Great for a packed lunch with some salad or cherry tomatoes.

SERVES 4–6

2 tablespoons olive oil
1 large onion, peeled, halved and very
    thinly sliced
250g new potatoes in their skins, cooked,
    cooled and thickly sliced
75g frozen baby broad beans or peas
6 eggs
2 tablespoons freshly chopped parsley
2 tablespoons freshly chopped mint
freshly ground black pepper

1. Heat the oil in a deep 20cm non-stick frying pan. Add the onion and cook over a medium heat until well softened – about 10 minutes. Add the potatoes and beans and cook, stirring, until warmed through.

2. Beat the eggs with the herbs and pepper and add to the pan. Stir carefully until the egg is half-set, then press the mixture lightly to flatten. Cook for a further 2–3 minutes until fairly firm, then loosen around the edges and slide the tortilla onto a plate.

3. Invert the pan over the top of the plate and return the tortilla to the pan. Cook the other side for 2–3 minutes until lightly golden. Serve warm or cold.

Per portion: 257 kcal, 15g fat, 3.6g sat fat, 0.13g sodium, 17g carbohydrate

Goat's Cheese, Pea and Dill Soufflé

A soufflé is much simpler to make than you might imagine. It's basically a rich cheese sauce with whisked egg whites folded in!

SERVES 4

25g cornflour
250ml semi-skimmed milk
½ teaspoon English mustard powder
¼ teaspoon cayenne pepper
¼ teaspoon ground nutmeg
100g frozen peas
150g mild soft goat's cheese
2 tablespoons freshly chopped dill
4 large eggs, separated

1. Butter a 1.8 litre soufflé dish. Preheat the oven to 200C°/400°F/gas mark 6 and set a baking tray on the oven shelf.

2. In a medium saucepan, mix the cornflour to a smooth paste with some of the milk then stir in the remainder. Add the spices and bring to a simmer, stirring all the time until thickened. Add the peas and simmer for 5 minutes, stirring occasionally.

3. Remove from the heat and stir in the cheese and dill followed by the egg yolks.

4. Whisk the egg whites until stiff then fold a spoonful into the cheese mixture. Fold this through the remaining egg whites until evenly combined and transfer to the soufflé dish. With the tip of your thumb make a narrow groove between the edge of the dish and the mixture; this helps the soufflé to rise evenly.

5. Bake on the hot oven tray for about 35 minutes until well risen and golden and just wobbly when very lightly shaken. Serve at once.

Per portion: 250 kcal, 16g fat, 4.2g sat fat, 0.14g sodium, 12g carbohydrate

Aubergine, Red Pepper, Rocket and Goat's Cheese Sandwiches

Char-grilled vegetables make a delicious and healthy filling for a sandwich – or try rolling them in a soft tortilla wrap. Always check labels; some medium-fat cheeses are much lower in calories than others!

SERVES 4

2 large red peppers, quartered and cored
1 large aubergine, cut lengthways in 12 slices
1 tablespoon olive oil
8 thin slices bread from a large seeded loaf
8 tablespoons soft medium-fat goat's cheese
50g rocket (or watercress)
lemon juice
freshly ground black pepper

1. Preheat the grill to high. Grill the pepper quarters skin-side up until well charred. Transfer to a covered bowl or plastic bag and leave for a few minutes to steam – this makes it easy to peel off the skin. Reserve any juices from the peppers.

2. Meanwhile, reduce the heat to medium. Brush the aubergine slices with the oil and grill for 5–7 minutes, until lightly charred and softened on both sides. Transfer to a plate and spoon over the juices from the peppers.

3. Spread the bread with the cheese and put a quarter of the pepper, aubergine and rocket on each of 4 of the slices. Season with lemon juice and pepper and top with the remaining slices.

Per portion: 400 kcal, 18g fat, 1.5g sat fat, 0.60g sodium, 42g carbohydrate

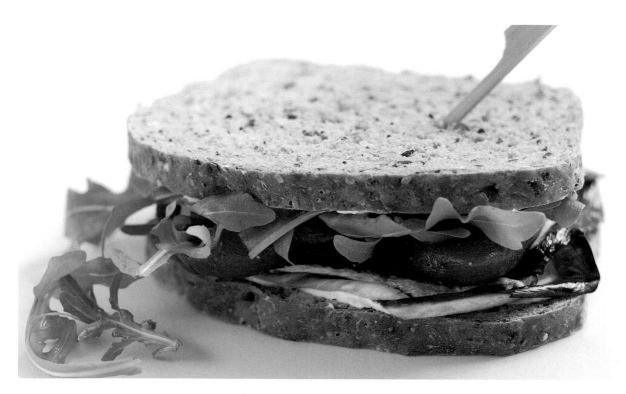

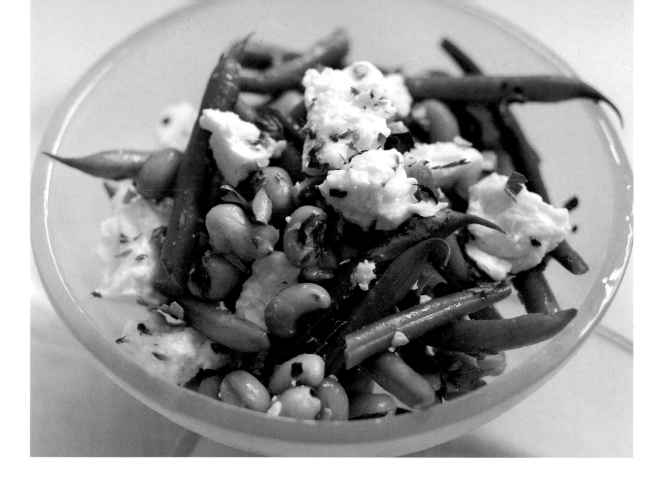

Warm Mixed Bean and Cheese Salad

There is a half-fat version of feta cheese available but it cannot be called 'feta' and so is referred to as Greek-style cheese. Try it for this recipe or alternatively choose a firm goat's cheese.

SERVES 4 as a starter / 2 as a main course

125g green beans, trimmed and cut in short lengths
400g tinned borlotti beans in water, drained and rinsed
1 tablespoon olive oil
2 tablespoons lemon juice
1 teaspoon dried oregano
½ teaspoon crushed dried chillies
3 tablespoons freshly chopped parsley
100g Greek-style cheese, crumbled
salad leaves, to serve (optional)

1. Steam the green beans for 4–5 minutes until just tender. Drain and immediately mix with the borlotti beans. Keep warm.

2. Whisk together all the remaining ingredients except the cheese using a fork. Fold through the beans then stir in the cheese.

3. Serve at once, piled on salad leaves, if wished.

Per portion (starter): 121 kcal, 5g fat, 0.4g sat fat, 0g sodium, 9g carbohydrate

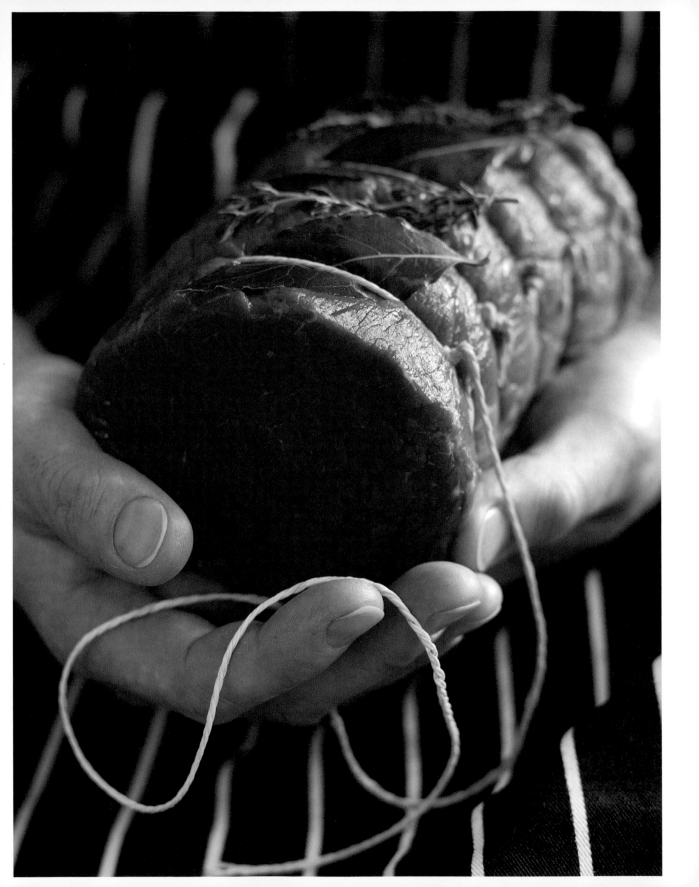

Meat and poultry

About meat and poultry

All types of meat and poultry and the offal from them such as liver and kidney consist mainly of protein and contain no carbohydrate, therefore they have a GI and GL of 0. They are important sources of protein, iron and zinc as well as of B vitamins.

The red meats are beef, pork and lamb. When buying, select fully trimmed lean meat in order to avoid extra fat and calories. This is especially true when buying minced meats.

Poultry includes chicken and turkey as well as duck and goose. Duck and goose are higher in fat so it is better to save them for special occasions. The fat on poultry is deposited mainly under the skin, so it is best to discard the skin either before or after cooking. Again, when buying minced poultry, check the pack for the fat content as sometimes the skin is used in the mince.

Offal is low in fat but liver is a rich source of cholesterol. Liver is a rich source of vitamin A but excessive amounts can be harmful to a growing foetus, so it is recommended that pregnant women do not eat it.

Sausages contain rusk but have a low GI and GL – look for good-quality sausages with a high percentage of meat. Their calorie content can be increased by frying so the best way to prepare them is by grilling, dry-frying or oven-baking.

Lean meat and bacon are not particularly high in fat and so can be enjoyed as part of a weight-loss diet. Limit yourself to a portion size of about 100g–150g.

Cooking

In order to keep the calorie content of meat and poultry low you should prepare it with as little extra fat or oil as possible. Simply use some oil or butter to prevent it sticking to the pan, applying it with a pastry brush or spray. This way a little goes a long way.

Remember too that batter and breadcrumbs soak up fat so avoid them if you are trying to lose weight.

Salt and meat

Fresh meat and poultry are naturally low in salt, but salt is added both as a preservative and to give the distinctive flavour when bacon, ham and sausages are made. This means that when a recipe includes bacon, ham or sausages, the sodium (salt) content will increase, so try to balance your day's food accordingly.

Fat content of raw meat and poultry (%)

Back bacon, lean	7
Beef, lean, average	5
Lamb, lean, average	8
Pork, lean, average	4
Chicken, light meat	1
Chicken, dark meat	3
Turkey, average	2

Fruity Beef Casserole

A rich and warming stew for a winter's day. Venison may be used to replace the beef. As with all casseroles, it is even better if left for a day to allow the flavours to mellow. Cool after making then chill in the fridge (this recipe will also freeze well). Reheat as required.

SERVES 6

1kg lean beef such as topside or silverside, cut in 3cm pieces
1 tablespoon cornflour
½ teaspoon ground black pepper
1 tablespoon vegetable oil
2 celery stalks, chopped
1 large onion, peeled and chopped
2 garlic cloves, peeled and finely chopped
2 sprigs of thyme
2 bay leaves
finely grated zest of 1 orange
1 tablespoon tomato purée
2 tablespoons redcurrant jelly
600ml beef stock
1 tablespoon Worcestershire sauce
12 ready-to-eat prunes
50g dried cranberries
200g jar of cooked chestnuts
250g button mushrooms, wiped

1. Preheat the oven to 130°C/275°F/gas mark 1.

2. Toss the meat in the cornflour and pepper. Heat the oil in a large flameproof casserole and brown the meat in batches. Return it all to the casserole.

3. Add the celery, onion, garlic, thyme, bay leaves, orange zest, tomato purée and redcurrant jelly. Stir in the stock and Worcestershire sauce and bring to a simmer.

4. Add the dried fruit, chestnuts and mushrooms and mix well. Once the stock is just simmering again, cover and transfer to the oven.

5. Cook for 2 hours until tender. Serve with a rough mash of white beans and celeriac or parsnip and some green beans.

Per portion: 378 kcal, 11g fat, 3.4g sat fat, 0.32g sodium, 33g carbohydrate

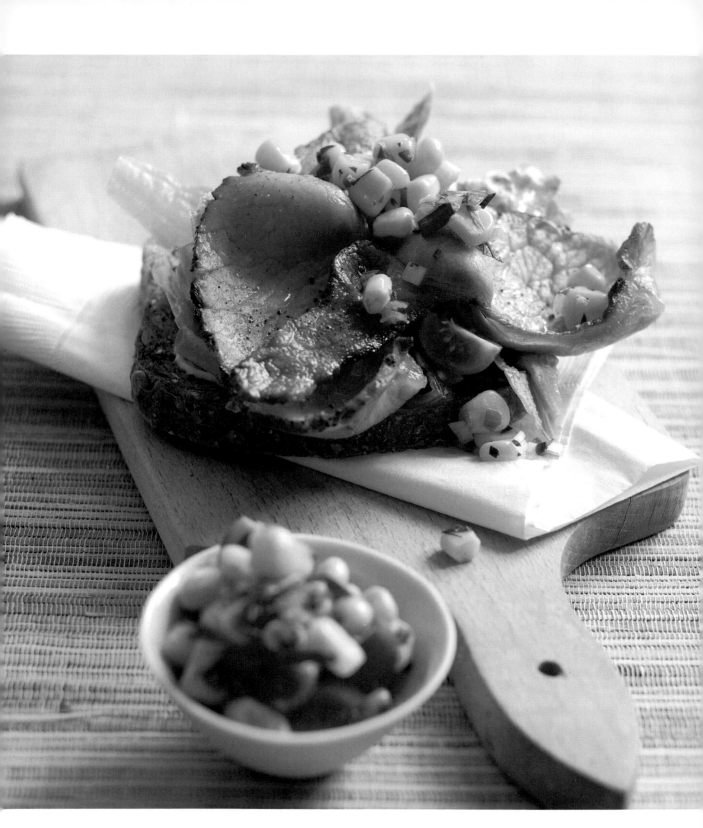

Open-Topped BLTs with Spicy Sweetcorn Salsa

This variation of the BLT has become a real favourite of mine!

SERVES 2

2 slices bread from a large seeded loaf, toasted
1 tablespoon reduced-calorie mayonnaise
50g iceberg lettuce, roughly torn
4 rashers very lean dry-cured back bacon, grilled
4 tablespoons Spicy Sweetcorn Salsa (see below)
freshly ground black pepper

1. Spread the toasted bread with the mayonnaise and divide the lettuce and bacon between the slices. Top with the salsa and finish off with a sprinkling of pepper.

Spicy Sweetcorn Salsa

MAKES 24 TABLESPOONS (12 SERVINGS)

250g frozen sweetcorn kernels
1 tablespoon raw cane brown sugar
1 tablespoon sherry vinegar (or wine vinegar or cider vinegar)
125g cherry tomatoes, quartered
2 large spring onions, finely chopped
1 red chilli, deseeded and finely chopped
1 tablespoon freshly chopped parsley
1 tablespoon freshly chopped coriander

1. Cook the sweetcorn according to the pack instructions, then drain thoroughly. While it is still warm, add the sugar and vinegar and mix to dissolve the sugar. Leave to cool then stir in the remaining ingredients.
   This will keep in the fridge for 2–3 days.

Per portion (including Spicy Sweetcorn Salsa): 288 kcal, 16g fat, 4.9g sat fat, 1.35g sodium, 19g carbohydrate

Aromatic Lamb Fillet

SERVES 4

1½ tablespoons finely chopped sage leaves
1½ tablespoons finely chopped thyme leaves
4 garlic cloves, finely chopped
4 pieces of neck of lamb fillet, about 125g each
1 teaspoon olive oil
150ml lamb or chicken stock

FOR THE BEANS

400g tinned flageolet beans, drained and rinsed
1 small red onion, finely chopped
2 bay leaves and 2 sprigs of thyme
250g cherry tomatoes, halved
3 tablespoons chopped flat-leafed parsley
3 tablespoons lamb or chicken stock
finely grated zest and juice of ½ lemon

1. Pound the sage, thyme, garlic and 3 table-spoons water to a thick paste, using a pestle and mortar or in a small food processor. Smear over the lamb fillets. Cover and leave in a cool place for at least 1 hour or refrigerate for up to 24 hours. Remove from the fridge 1 hour before cooking.

2. Preheat the oven to 180°C/350°F/gas mark 4. Heat a frying pan until hot and add the oil. Sear the lamb for 2 minutes on each side, then transfer to the oven for a further 5–10 minutes, depending on how pink you like it. Leave to rest for 5 minutes.

3. Put the beans, red onion, bay leaves, thyme, tomatoes and parsley in a saucepan with the stock. Simmer for 3–4 minutes, stirring. Add the lemon zest and juice and season with black pepper.

4. Add the stock to any meat juices that have gathered in the pan. Heat for a couple of minutes, scraping up any sediment from the pan. Season with pepper. To serve, spoon the bean mixture onto warm serving plates. Slice the lamb and pile on top then drizzle with the pan juices.

Per portion: 299 kcal, 12g fat, 4.6g sat fat, 0.44g sodium, 15g carbohydrate

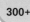

Lamb Chump Steaks with Mint Mechoui

The combination of beating the meat and marinating it keeps the lamb really tender. Serve this classic combination with courgettes and baby new potatoes.

SERVES 4

4 lean lamb chump steaks, about 100–125g each
15g fresh mint leaves, chopped
juice of 1 lemon
2 garlic cloves, peeled and crushed
1 tablespoon ground coriander
1 teaspoon paprika
1 teaspoon ground cumin
½ teaspoon freshly ground black pepper
½ teaspoon cayenne pepper
fresh mint leaves to garnish

1. Wipe the meat with a damp cloth. Using a meat mallet or rolling pin, beat each piece of meat to flatten it to about twice its size.

2. Combine the remaining ingredients with 1 tablespoon cold water.

3. Spoon this mixture over the meat, turning the meat well to coat completely. Cover and marinate in a cool place for at least 1 hour or preferably in the fridge for 24–48 hours. Remove from the fridge 1 hour before cooking.

4. Preheat the grill to maximum and cook the lamb steaks for 3–5 minutes each side, depending on whether you like the meat pink or well cooked. Serve garnished with extra mint leaves.

**Per portion: 205 kcal, 11g fat, 4.4g sat fat,
0.10g sodium, 2g carbohydrate**

Lamb Curry with Chick Peas and Spinach

As with all curries and stews, this dish is best prepared 1–2 days in advance to allow the flavours to mellow. Once cool, store in the fridge and add the spinach when reheating.

SERVES 4

100g dried chick peas
500g lean shoulder of lamb, cut into 2cm pieces
300g 0% fat Greek yogurt
400g tinned chopped tomatoes
2 teaspoons cornflour
1 teaspoon ground turmeric
1 teaspoon ground coriander
½ teaspoon ground nutmeg
½ teaspoon ground cinnamon
1 onion, peeled and grated
1 tablespoon freshly grated ginger
3 garlic cloves, peeled and crushed
finely grated zest of 1 orange
2 green chillies, deseeded and finely chopped
175g baby spinach leaves

1. Generously cover the chick peas with cold water and leave to soak overnight. Combine all the remaining ingredients except the spinach in a flameproof casserole and leave overnight in the fridge.

2. Preheat the oven to 150°C/300°F/gas mark 2. Stir the lamb mixture well then bring to a simmer on top of the stove. Drain and rinse the chick peas and add to the casserole. Cover and transfer to the oven, then cook for 2 hours. Check and stir after 1 hour – you should not need to add any extra water.

3. Just before serving, bring the curry back to a simmer on top of the stove and stir in the spinach, a little at a time, until well wilted. Serve with brown basmati rice, mixed with wild rice.

**Per portion: 374 kcal, 12g fat, 4.6g sat fat,
0.20g sodium, 27g carbohydrate**

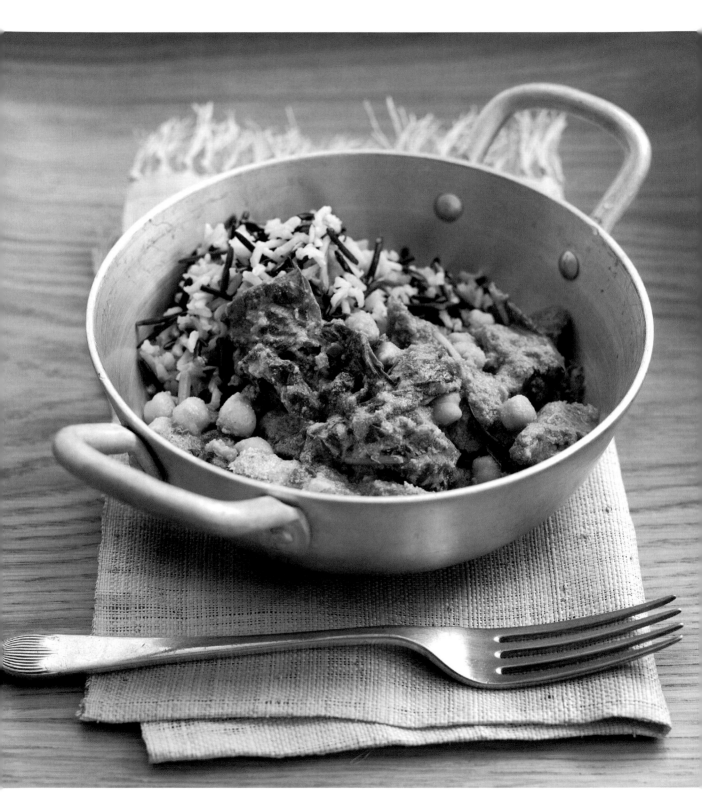

Chicken Livers with Moroccan Spices

Fresh chicken livers are available from butchers and some supermarkets.

SERVES 2

400g chicken livers
1 teaspoon ground cumin
½ teaspoon ground coriander
¼ teaspoon chilli powder
¼ teaspoon paprika
¼ teaspoon ground black pepper
2 garlic cloves, peeled and crushed
1 tablespoon olive oil
1 tablespoon freshly chopped mint
1 tablespoon freshly chopped coriander
juice of ½ small lemon
salad leaves with carrot ribbons, to serve

1. Clean the chicken livers, discarding all membrane and sinew. Rinse and pat dry with kitchen paper then cut into bite-size pieces.

2. Mix the spices, garlic and oil and toss the chicken livers in the mixture to coat evenly. Cover and marinate in a cool place for at least 30 minutes or in the fridge for up to 24 hours. Remove from the fridge 30 minutes before cooking.

3. Heat a dry wok or large non-stick frying pan over a high heat. Add the chicken livers with all the marinade and stir-fry for 3–5 minutes, depending on whether you like the livers pink or well cooked.

4. Add the herbs and lemon juice and serve at once on top of a bed of salad leaves and carrot ribbons.

Per portion: 239 kcal, 11g fat, 2.2g sat fat, 0.16g sodium, 1g carbohydrate

Lamb's Liver with Shallots and Balsamic Vinegar

A dash of balsamic vinegar cuts through the richness of the liver – use lemon juice as an alternative.

SERVES 2

200g lamb's liver, thinly sliced
1 tablespoon olive oil
2 sprigs of fresh rosemary
2 large shallots, peeled, halved lengthways
    and thinly sliced
2 teaspoons balsamic vinegar
4 tablespoons fresh beef stock
freshly ground black pepper
2 stems of vine cherry tomatoes, lightly grilled,
    to serve

1. Wash the liver and pat dry on kitchen paper. Remove any membrane and sinew. Turn the liver in 2 teaspoons olive oil and season generously with pepper.

2. Heat a dry non-stick frying pan over a high heat, add the liver and sear for 1 minute each side. Remove from the pan and keep warm.

3. Add the remaining oil to the pan with the rosemary sprigs and shallots and cook quickly just to soften slightly. Stir in the balsamic vinegar and then the stock. Heat gently then spoon over the liver. Serve at once with the grilled vine tomatoes and some steamed green beans or broccoli.

Per portion: 193 kcal, 12g fat, 2.5g sat fat, 0.15g sodium, 1g carbohydrate

Butternut Squash and Sausage Casserole

Autumn brings lots of different types of pumpkin and squash, so feel free to use other varieties.

SERVES 4

1 tablespoon olive oil
454g pack reduced-fat sausages, cut in
    3cm chunks
1 onion, peeled and roughly chopped
2 garlic cloves, peeled and roughly chopped
1 red pepper, deseeded and roughly chopped
1 red chilli, deseeded and finely diced
1 teaspoon fresh thyme leaves
1 teaspoon paprika
1 butternut squash (about 800g prepared weight)
    peeled, deseeded and cut into 4cm chunks
400g tinned chopped tomatoes
410g tinned butter beans in water, drained
    and rinsed
freshly ground black pepper

1. Grill the sausage chunks until brown on all sides. Set aside.

2. Add the onion, garlic, pepper, chilli and thyme to a large flameproof casserole and cook over a medium heat until the onion starts to soften. Add 1–2 tablespoons water as necessary to stop the ingredients sticking. Stir in the paprika and return the sausages to the casserole. Mix well and cook for 1–2 minutes.

3. Add the squash, tomatoes and 100ml water and bring to a simmer. Cover and bake for 30 minutes. Stir in the beans and bake for a further 15 minutes. Season to taste with pepper and serve with steamed green beans or cabbage wedges.

Per portion: 349 kcal, 7g fat, 0.5g sat fat, 0.71g sodium, 49g carbohydrate

Paprika Turkey in Pitta Pockets

Turkey and chicken absorb strong flavours extremely well. This is an easy snack that will suit all the family.

SERVES 4

1 tablespoon Worcestershire sauce
1 tablespoon clear honey
1 tablespoon paprika
1 tablespoon wholegrain mustard
400g turkey escalopes (or chicken breast fillet),
    cut in strips
1 tablespoon vegetable oil
150g 0% fat Greek yogurt
4 pitta breads, warmed
shredded lettuce, watercress or baby spinach
    leaves, to serve
shredded red pepper, to serve

1. Mix together the Worcestershire sauce, honey, paprika and mustard then combine with the turkey. Cover and marinate in a cool place for at least 1 hour or in the fridge for up to 24 hours. Remove from the fridge 1 hour before cooking.

2. Heat the oil in a non-stick frying pan, add the turkey with all the marinade and fry over a high heat for 5 minutes until cooked through. Remove from the heat and fold the yogurt through.

3. Split the pittas and stuff each with some salad leaves, red pepper and a quarter of the turkey mixture. Serve at once.

Per portion: 421 kcal, 5g fat, 0.9g sat fat, 0.56g sodium, 59g carbohydrate

Roast Garlic Chicken with Lemon and Macadamias

This one-bake dish is simple to make and perfect for entertaining during the week.

SERVES 4

8 skinless chicken thighs – about 850g
freshly ground black pepper
1 tablespoon macadamia oil (or vegetable oil)
12 unpeeled garlic cloves
2 tablespoons macadamia nuts
500g sugar snap peas
finely grated zest and juice of 1 lemon

1. Preheat the oven to 220°C/425°F/gas mark 7. Wash the chicken and pat dry with kitchen paper. Season with pepper.

2. Heat the oil in a non-stick roasting tin and turn the pieces of chicken in it. Add the garlic cloves and nuts and roast for 25 minutes.

3. Meanwhile, blanch the sugar snap peas for 1 minute. Drain thoroughly.

4. Spoon the sugar snap peas around the chicken, sprinkle with lemon zest and juice, then return to the oven for 5 minutes. Serve at once.

Per portion: 308 kcal, 12g fat, 2.3g sat fat, 0.18g sodium, 9g carbohydrate

Thai Green Chicken Curry

Do buy an authentic green curry paste from an Asian shop if possible. It makes all the difference to the finished curry. One tablespoon of paste will give a mild flavour, two will add a 'kick'! I like to have a thin sauce for this curry to ensure there are plenty of juices to go with the rice.

SERVES 4

1–2 tablespoons Thai green curry paste
1 teaspoon vegetable oil
2 stalks lemongrass, tender inner part only, finely chopped
2 fresh (or dried) kaffir lime leaves, finely shredded
400ml tinned reduced-fat coconut milk
500g skinless, boneless chicken thighs (about 6 thighs), cut into bite-sized pieces
100g baby corn, sliced
50g green beans, cut into 2cm pieces
50g frozen peas
4 tablespoons freshly chopped coriander leaves and stalks
2 large green chillies, deseeded and finely chopped
4 tablespoons freshly torn basil leaves
1 tablespoon fish sauce (nam pla)
fresh lime, to squeeze

1. Fry the curry paste in the oil over a low heat, stirring, for 2–3 minutes. Add the lemongrass, lime leaves and coconut milk and simmer for 5 minutes.

2. Add the chicken, vegetables, coriander, chillies and 200ml water, and bring to a simmer. Simmer, uncovered, for 15 minutes.

3. Just before serving, stir in the basil leaves and fish sauce and add a squeeze of fresh lime, to taste. Serve with rice.

Per portion: 287 kcal, 13g fat, 0.5g sat fat, 0.44g sodium, 9g carbohydrate

Pot-Roast Chicken

As the name suggests this is a one-pot meal – all you need is a large flameproof casserole to hold the chicken and its accompanying vegetables. Chicken skin is high in calories so ideally you shouldn't eat it!

SERVES 4

1.5kg corn-fed chicken
1 tablespoon vegetable oil
1 onion, peeled and roughly chopped
2 garlic cloves, peeled and finely chopped
2 celery stalks, cut into 3cm chunks
2 large carrots, cut into 3cm chunks
12 new potatoes
1 tablespoon fresh thyme leaves
2 bay leaves
400g tinned chopped tomatoes
1 tablespoon Worcestershire sauce
300ml chicken stock
250g small broccoli florets
125g frozen peas
125g frozen baby broad beans
50g baby spinach leaves
freshly ground black pepper

1. Preheat the oven to 190°C/375°F/gas mark 5. Wash the chicken inside and out, pat dry with kitchen paper and tie in a neat shape with string.

2. Heat the oil in a flameproof casserole and brown the chicken on all sides. Discard the excess fat from the casserole. Set the chicken breast-side up and add the onion, garlic, celery, carrots, potatoes, thyme and bay leaves. Pour in the chopped tomatoes, Worcestershire sauce and stock and bring to a simmer.

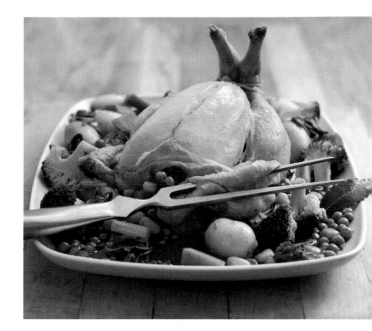

3. Cover and cook in the centre of the oven for 1 hour until the chicken is cooked (test the thickest part of the thigh with a skewer – the juices should run clear) and the vegetables are just tender.

4. Remove the chicken from the casserole and set aside in a warm place to rest. Add the green vegetables to the casserole, season with pepper and bring to a simmer on top of the stove. Cover then cook for 10 minutes.

5. Carve the chicken, discarding all the skin and serve with the vegetables and tomato broth.

Per portion: 401 kcal, 10g fat, 2.8g sat fat, 0.51g sodium, 40g carbohydrate

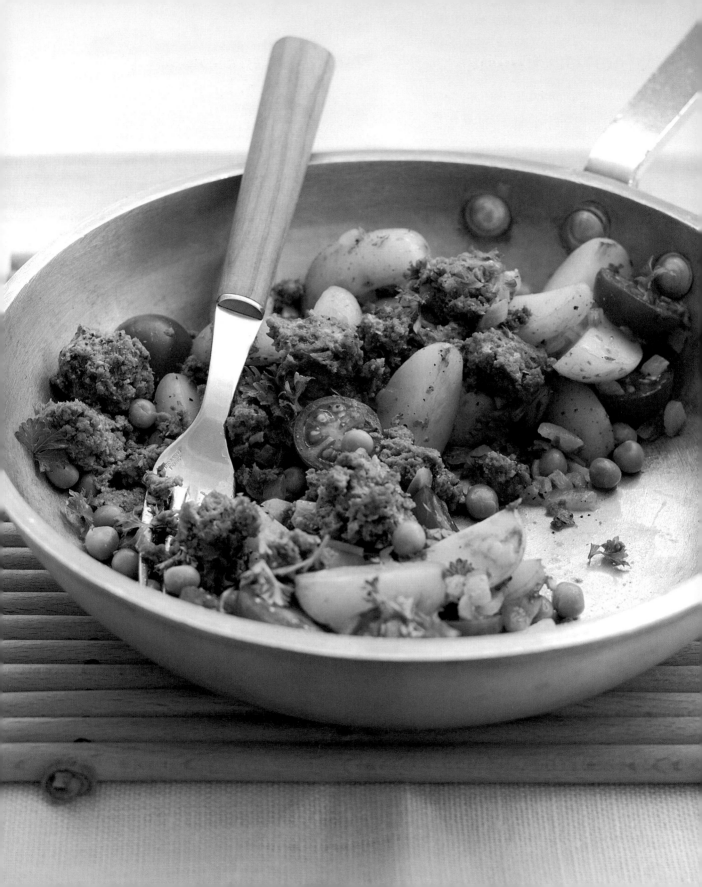

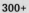

Corned Beef Hash

An easy brunch or supper dish that uses basic ingredients.

SERVES 4

500g small new potatoes
1 tablespoon vegetable oil
1 large onion, peeled and finely chopped
340g tinned corned beef, diced
200g frozen peas, blanched
200g cherry tomatoes, halved
4 tablespoons semi-skimmed milk
4 tablespoons freshly chopped parsley
freshly ground black pepper

1. Wash and quarter the potatoes lengthways then steam until tender – about 10 minutes.

2. Heat the oil in a large non-stick frying pan and cook the onion over a gentle heat for about 10 minutes until lightly golden. Add the potatoes to the pan and cook for a further 5 minutes until lightly golden. Stir in the corned beef and cook for 1–2 minutes.

3. Stir in the peas and tomatoes. Moisten with the milk and add the parsley. Season with pepper and stir until heated through. Serve at once.

Per portion: 352 kcal, 13g fat, 5.6g sat fat, 0.76g sodium, 32g carbohydrate

Pork, Prune and Apple Hot Pot

SERVES 4

½ small celeriac, peeled (about 175g peeled weight)
1 medium sweet potato (about 175g)
1 medium cooking apple, quartered, cored and thinly sliced
1 large onion (about 175g) peeled, halved and thinly sliced
75g small ready-to-eat prunes
freshly ground black pepper
2 bay leaves
300ml fresh chicken stock
1 tablespoon wholegrain mustard
4 pork steaks (about 125g each) trimmed of excess fat
freshly chopped parsley, to serve

1. Preheat the oven to 180°C/350°F/gas mark 4.

2. Thinly slice the celeriac and sweet potato and place in a large saucepan. Cover with cold water and bring to the boil. Drain thoroughly.

3. Layer the celeriac, sweet potato, apple, onion and prunes in an ovenproof baking dish, seasoning with pepper and adding the bay leaves as you layer. Bring the stock to the boil in a pan and stir in the mustard.

4. Set the pork steaks on top of the vegetables and season with pepper. Pour the hot stock over, cover with foil and bake for 1 hour.

5. Remove the foil, spoon the stock over the meat and continue to cook for a further 15 minutes. Sprinkle with parsley and serve with a green vegetable such as brussels sprouts, green beans or broccoli.

Per portion: 263 kcal, 6g fat, 1.8g sat fat, 0.48g sodium, 23g carbohydrate

Pork Fillet Stroganoff

Using yogurt instead of double cream dramatically reduces the calories in this dish – the cornflour is added to stabilise the yogurt as it's warmed. Serve with noodles or brown basmati rice and a green vegetable or salad.

SERVES 4

1 tablespoon vegetable oil
500g pork tenderloin, cut in thick strips about 1cm wide
15g unsalted butter
1 onion, peeled and finely chopped
250g closed cup mushrooms, wiped and thickly sliced
1 teaspoon fresh thyme leaves
1 tablespoon Worcestershire sauce
1 tablespoon Dijon mustard
1 teaspoon paprika
150g 0% fat Greek yogurt
1 tablespoon cornflour mixed with 100ml cold water
freshly ground black pepper

1. Preheat a large non-stick frying pan over a high heat and add the oil. Add the pork and stir fry for 2–3 minutes until lightly browned. Remove from the pan.

2. Add the butter to the pan, then the onion, mushrooms and thyme and pan fry until just softened. Stir in the Worcestershire sauce, mustard and paprika.

3. Return the pork with its juices to the pan and mix well. Combine the yogurt and cornflour mixture and fold through the meat to warm through. Season with pepper.
    You may like to add a little extra water for a thinner sauce or another tub of yogurt for a creamier sauce.

Per portion: 275 kcal, 12g fat, 4.1g sat fat, 0.30g sodium, 10g carbohydrate

Asian Beef Salad

The fresh flavours and crisp texture of the vegetables balance the richness of the steak. You can also try it with chicken or duck breast fillets, altering the cooking times accordingly. Always allow the meat to come to room temperature for 30 minutes before cooking and leave to rest for at least 5 minutes after cooking for the juices to settle.

SERVES 4

2 x sirloin steaks, about 200g each, trimmed of all fat
1 large red chilli, deseeded and finely chopped
1 large garlic clove, peeled and very thinly sliced
1 tablespoon reduced-salt soy sauce
1 tablespoon fish sauce (*nam pla*)
juice of 1 lime
½ teaspoon golden caster sugar
1 red pepper, cored and finely shredded
1 yellow pepper, cored and finely shredded
4 spring onions. finely shredded
½ cucumber, quartered lengthways and thickly sliced
2 tablespoons roughly chopped fresh mint
2 tablespoons roughly chopped fresh coriander
50g raw peanuts
1 tablespoon sesame seeds

1. Preheat a dry non-stick frying pan over a high heat and add a tiny knob of the fat trimmed from one of the steaks. Add the steaks and sear for 1–1½ minutes on each side, then leave to rest on a plate.

2. Combine all the remaining ingredients in a salad bowl and mix well.

3. Thinly slice the steaks and add to the salad with all the meat juices. Serve at once.

Per portion: 256 kcal, 12g fat, 3.3g sat fat, 0.20g sodium, 8g carbohydrate

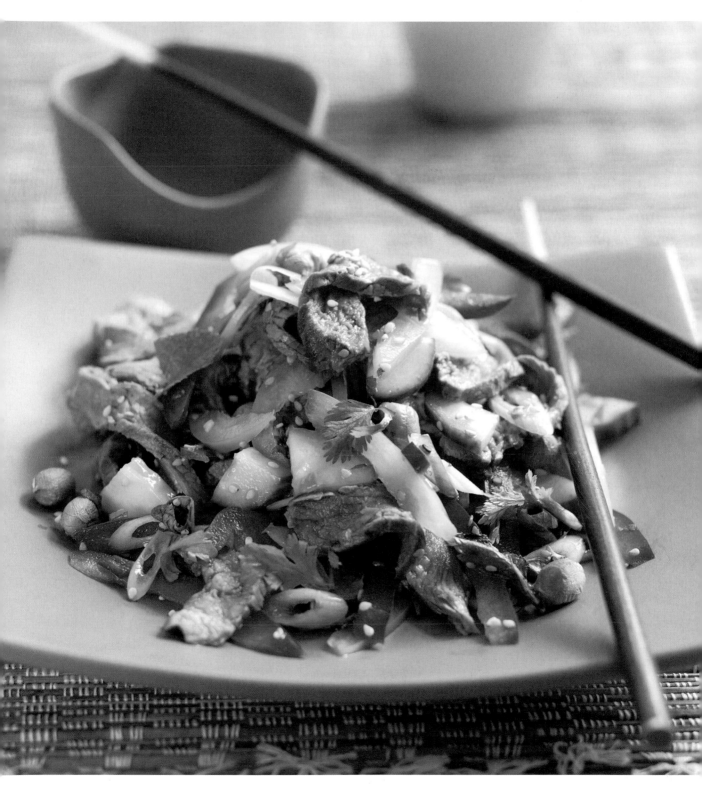

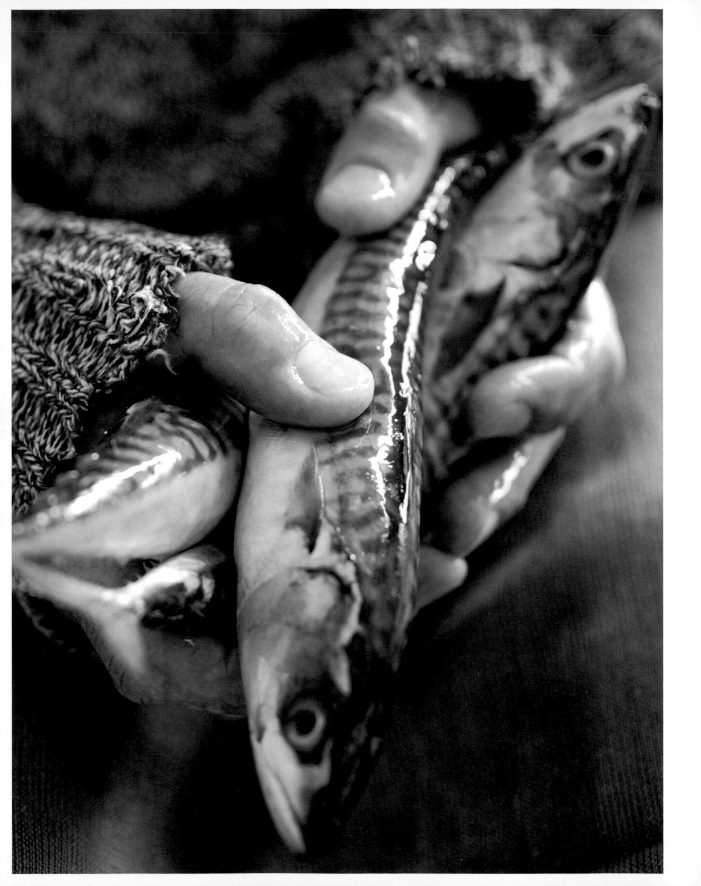

Fish and shellfish

About fish and shellfish

Like meat, fish and shellfish contain no carbohydrate so they have a GI and GL of 0. The main contribution they make to the diet is that they provide protein, some iron – in the more easily absorbed haem form – and zinc, also in a readily absorbed form.

Fish and shellfish contain varying amounts of fat and cholesterol. As with all protein foods, they provide calories so try not eat over-large portions.

Fresh fish is wonderful for flavour but frozen fish is also a good source of nutrients.

White fish
White fish is particularly low in fat, containing only 1–2 per cent. They are therefore low in calories as well.

White fish includes:

Cod	Pollock
Haddock	Sole
Halibut	Whiting
Plaice	

A 150g portion, steamed, provides about 120 kcal as well as protein, iodine, B vitamins and the antioxidant mineral selenium.

Oily or fatty fish
As the name implies, these fish have a greater fat content than white fish – an average of 15 per cent. They also contain vitamin D. They are especially important as they provide omega 3 and omega 6 fatty acids, which seem to offer some protection against coronary heart disease.

Fatty fish include:

Anchovies	Salmon
Herring	Sardine
Mackerel	Trout
Pilchards	Tuna
	Whitebait

Tinned and smoked versions of these fish may have a higher sodium (salt) content than their fresh equivalents. Use them to add variety to your diet but wherever possible, choose tinned fish in water. If you can only find fish in brine or oil, wash it well in a sieve under a running tap.

Shellfish
These include a wide variety of sea molluscs and crustaceans. Although shellfish are low in fat they can be a rich source of cholesterol, so if you have a raised cholesterol level, you should avoid eating them too often.

Examples of molluscs are:

Clams	Scallops
Cockles	Whelks
Mussels	Winkles
Oysters	

Oysters are a rich source of zinc. When buying scallops, choose diver-caught ones as this method does less damage to the seabed.

Examples of crustaceans are:

Crayfish	Prawns
Lobster	Shrimps

It is also worth considering produce from sustainable fisheries, for example. North Atlantic stocks of salmon and North Sea cod are currently very low and choosing organic farmed fish may be a sensible alternative.

Garlic Chilli Prawns with Papaya

Raw prawns take only 2–3 minutes to cook so be careful not to overcook them; they are ready when they turn pink. Serve with freshly cooked rice or on salad leaves.

SERVES 2

2 teaspoons olive oil
2 garlic cloves, peeled and chopped
200g medium raw prawns, shelled
½ teaspoon paprika
1 small dried chilli, crumbled
1 ripe papaya, quartered, deseeded, peeled and
   thickly sliced
juice of ½ lemon or of 1 lime
2 tablespoons freshly chopped parsley
freshly ground black pepper

1. Heat the oil in a large non-stick frying pan and sauté the garlic over a medium heat for 1 minute.

2. Add the prawns, paprika and chilli and stir-fry for 2 minutes.

3. Add the remaining ingredients and stir carefully for 1 minute. Serve at once.

Per portion: 150 kcal, 4g fat, 0.5g sat fat, 0.24g sodium, 9g carbohydrate

Cod, Prawn and Sweetcorn Chowder

SERVES 4–6

1 tablespoon vegetable oil
2 onions, peeled and chopped
250g new potatoes, diced
1 bay leaf
few sprigs of fresh thyme
900ml fish stock
2 red peppers, deseeded and diced
100g frozen peas
100g frozen sweetcorn
410g tinned cannellini beans in water, drained
   and rinsed
2 tablespoons potato flour or cornflour
300ml semi-skimmed milk
350g cod fillet, cut in 3cm pieces
100g raw peeled prawns
freshly ground black pepper
2 tablespoons freshly chopped parsley
2 tablespoons freshly snipped chives

1. Heat the oil in a large saucepan, add the onions and cook until soft and translucent – you may need to add a tablespoon of stock to prevent them sticking. Add the potatoes, bay leaf and thyme and mix well.

2. Pour in the stock and bring to a simmer. Simmer, covered, for 15 minutes then add all the vegetables and bring to a simmer.

3. In a bowl, mix the potato flour with a little of the milk to a smooth paste then add the rest of the milk and stir into the pan. Add the cod and simmer for 3 minutes then stir in the prawns and simmer for a further 2 minutes.

4. Season to taste with pepper, stir in the herbs and serve.

Per portion: 374 kcal, 7g fat, 1.5g sat fat, 0.46g sodium, 48g carbohydrate

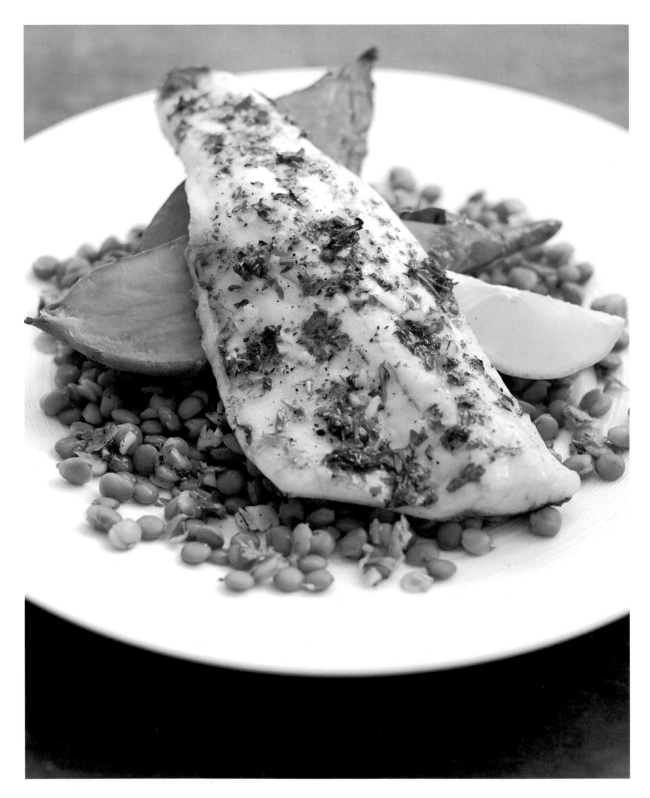

Grilled Seabass Fillets with Salmoriglio and Lentils

Based on a Sicilian recipe which usually uses a lot more olive oil, this fresher version goes perfectly with seabass but is also suited to other thin fish fillets such as halibut, pollock, plaice or lemon sole. Cooking times will vary according to the thickness of the fish. Serve with broccoli and baked sweet potatoes in their jackets.

SERVES 2

1½ teaspoons dried oregano
2 small garlic cloves, peeled and crushed
4 teaspoons olive oil
2 tablespoons lemon juice
1 tablespoon freshly chopped parsley
2 fillets seabass, about 150g each
300g tinned green lentils, drained and rinsed
freshly ground black pepper

1. Make a marinade by whisking together the oregano, garlic, olive oil, lemon juice, parsley and plenty of pepper with 1 tablespoon water.

2. Wash the fish fillets, pat dry on kitchen paper, then lay them on a plate and spoon over half the marinade. Cover and leave in the fridge for 1–2 hours.

3. Preheat the grill to maximum and grill the fillets, skin-side down, for 5–6 minutes until just cooked through – the flesh should be white when tested with the point of a small knife.

4. Meanwhile, warm the lentils with the remaining marinade. Spoon onto warmed plates and top with the seabass. Serve at once.

Per portion: 278 kcal, 10g fat, 1.6g sat fat, 0.49g sodium, 12g carbohydrate

Seared Tuna on Warm Pak Choi with Mustard Seed, Ginger and Lime Dressing

Tuna dries out quickly if cooked for too long. Ideally it should be pink in the middle, much like a steak.

SERVES 4

4 tuna steaks, about 125g each
1 tablespoon walnut oil
1 garlic clove, peeled and thinly sliced
1 tablespoon freshly grated ginger
½ teaspoon black mustard seeds
400g pak choi, sliced
1 tablespoon reduced-salt soy sauce

MARINADE
2 teaspoons clear honey
1 small red chilli, deseeded and finely chopped
finely grated zest and juice of 1 lime

1. Mix all the ingredients for the marinade. Wipe the tuna, turn it in the marinade, then cover and leave for at least 1 hour. Remove from the fridge 1 hour before cooking .

2. Heat 1 teaspoon walnut oil in a large non-stick frying pan over a high heat. Remove the tuna steaks from the marinade and pat dry with kitchen paper. Reserve the juices. Add the tuna to the pan and sear for 1 minute each side. Remove from the pan and leave to rest while you cook the pak choi.

3. Heat the remaining oil in the pan, add the garlic, ginger and mustard seeds and cook for 30 seconds. Stir in the pak choi and stir-fry for 2 minutes. Add the reserved marinade and simmer for 1–2 minutes. Stir in the soy sauce and serve at once with the tuna.

Per portion: 216 kcal, 9g fat, 1.8g sat fat, 0.18g sodium, 4g carbohydrate

Haddock with a Horseradish Herb Crust

When horseradish is not in season you can buy grated horseradish in jars from a good delicatessen or supermarket.

SERVES 4

6 tablespoons fresh wholegrain breadcrumbs
2 tablespoons freshly grated horseradish
1 tablespoon freshly chopped parsley
1 tablespoon freshly chopped thyme leaves
1 teaspoon freshly chopped rosemary leaves
2 spring onions, finely chopped
2 teaspoons unsalted butter, softened
4 pieces haddock or pollock fillet or halibut
    steaks, about 125–150g each
freshly ground black pepper
lemon wedges, to serve

1. Preheat the oven to 180°C/350°F/gas mark 4.

2. Combine the first seven ingredients in a bowl and season with pepper. Wash the fish and pat dry on kitchen paper. Set in an ovenproof dish.

3. Press the herb mixture evenly on top and pour 4 tablespoons water around the fish. Bake, uncovered, for about 20 minutes depending on the thickness of the fish. When tested, the fish should be white and no longer translucent.

4. Serve with wedges of lemon to squeeze. Good accompaniments are steamed new potatoes and a green vegetable such as green beans, peas or broccoli.

Per portion: 197 kcal, 3g fat, 1.5g sat fat, 0.18g sodium, 13g carbohydrate

Prawn and Noodle Salad with Peanut Dressing

Soak beansprouts in cold water for 5 minutes then drain thoroughly – it really improves their crunch! You can replace the rice noodles with other noodles such as soba (buckwheat).

SERVES 4

100g thin rice noodles
250g cooked peeled prawns
150g beansprouts
150g sugar snap peas, roughly shredded
4 spring onions, shredded
2 tablespoons freshly chopped coriander
1 tablespoon sesame seeds, toasted in a dry
    frying pan

DRESSING
75g coarse peanut butter
1 tablespoon reduced-salt soy sauce
1 tablespoon clear honey
½ teaspoon crushed garlic
1 red chilli, deseeded and finely chopped
2 tablespoons rice vinegar

1. For the dressing, mix all the ingredients together in a bowl with 2 tablespoons hot water from the kettle.

2. Put the noodles in a large heatproof bowl and cover with boiling water from the kettle. Leave to soak for 5 minutes then drain thoroughly and refresh in cold water. Drain thoroughly once more.

3. Combine all the remaining ingredients in a large bowl, add the drained noodles, stir the dressing through and serve at once.

Per portion: 308 kcal, 12g fat, 2.7g sat fat, 0.31g sodium, 30g carbohydrate

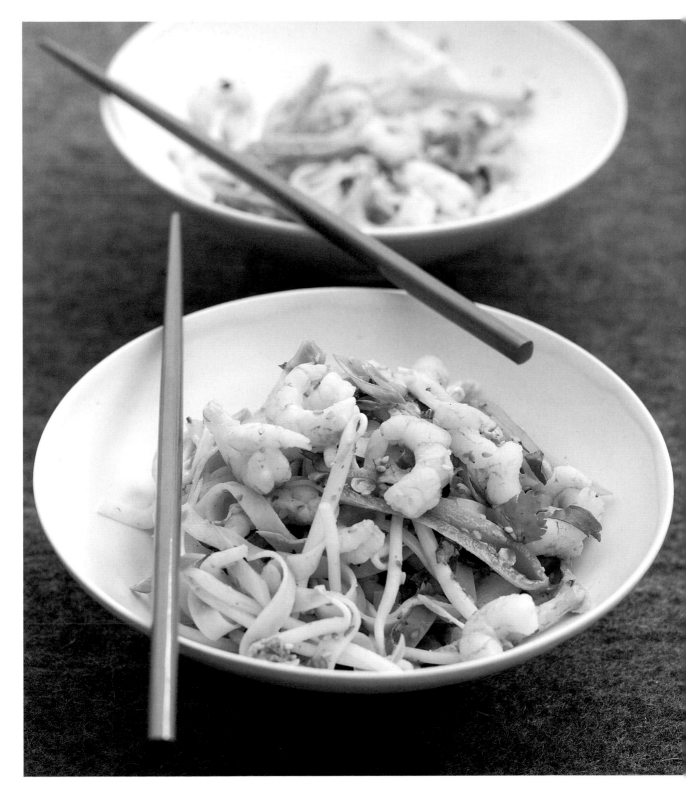

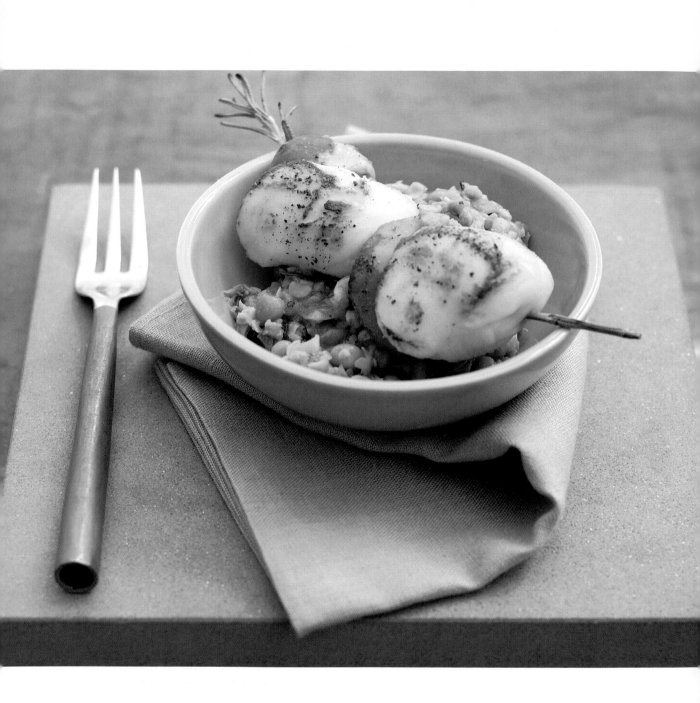

Seared Scallops with Crushed Minted Peas

The secret to cooking scallops is to turn them in olive oil to moisten, then get the pan very hot before you add them. For a special presentation thread them onto rosemary stalks before cooking.

SERVES 2

4 large fresh scallops (or 8 small ones)
1 teaspoon olive oil
freshly ground black pepper

PEAS
15g unsalted butter
6 spring onions, thinly sliced
175g frozen peas
150ml vegetable stock
2 tablespoons freshly chopped mint leaves

1. Wash the scallops and pat dry on kitchen paper. Turn them in the oil and season with pepper. Set aside while you prepare the peas.

2. Melt the butter in a saucepan, add the onions and soften for 1–2 minutes over a medium heat. Add the peas and stock and bring to the boil. Reduce the heat and simmer, uncovered, for 5 minutes. Stir the mint through then pulse in a food-processor until roughly crushed. Return to the pan, season with pepper and keep warm.

3. Put a small non-stick frying pan over a high heat. When hot, add the scallops and sear for 1–2 minutes on each side (no longer or they will become tough). Remove from the pan and serve at once on top of the crushed peas. This is delicious with chunky oven-baked chips.

Per portion: 238 kcal, 10g fat, 4.6g sat fat, 0.74g sodium, 12g carbohydrate

Sugar and Spice Salmon with Char-Grilled Corn Salsa

This salsa really needs to be made when fresh corn cobs are available but in an emergency, replace with 100g frozen or tinned sweetcorn kernels. The salmon pieces look like 'lollipops' which might entice children to eat them!

SERVES 2

2 pieces salmon fillet, about 125g each, skinned
2 teaspoons raw cane soft brown sugar
½ teaspoon dried mixed herbs
¼ teaspoon chilli powder

CORN SALSA
1 large corn on the cob
½ red pepper, deseeded
1½ tablespoons freshly chopped coriander
1 tablespoon red onion, peeled and
    finely chopped
2 teaspoons pickled jalapeño chilli,
    finely chopped

1. For the salsa, char-grill the corn cob and the pepper half, either directly over a gas flame or under a preheated grill. Leave to cool then cut the kernels off the cob. Skin and finely chop the red pepper. Mix the corn and pepper with the remaining salsa ingredients. Cover and set aside.

2. Rinse the salmon and pat dry on kitchen. Cut each piece into 4 thin strips and thread a skewer through each one. Mix the sugar, herbs and chilli powder and lightly sprinkle the mixture on both sides of the salmon.

3. Preheat the grill to high and cook the salmon 'lollipops' for 1 minute each side. Serve with the salsa and a wedge of lime to squeeze.

Per portion: 351 kcal, 20g fat, 2.4g sat fat, 0.88g sodium, 17g carbohydrate

Italian-Style Roast Monkfish Tail with Warm Spinach Salad

Roasting monkfish on the bone keeps it moist.

SERVES 2

1 small monkfish tail, about 300g
1 teaspoon olive oil
2 teaspoons freshly chopped rosemary leaves
freshly ground black pepper
2 plum tomatoes, halved

SPINACH
1 teaspoon olive oil
1 tablespoon pine nuts
1 garlic clove, peeled and sliced
225g baby spinach
1 tablespoon raisins
lemon juice

1. Preheat the oven to 220°C/425°F/gas mark 7. Remove any membrane from the fish then wash and pat dry on kitchen paper. Mix together the olive oil and rosemary, season generously with pepper and use to coat the fish. Place in a small roasting tin with the tomatoes and cook in the oven, uncovered, for about 20 minutes until the flesh is firm and white and no longer translucent when tested with a small sharp knife.

2. Meanwhile, prepare the spinach. Heat the oil in a frying pan and pan fry the pine nuts and garlic until golden. Add the spinach leaves, a handful at a time, until just wilted. Add the raisins and season to taste with lemon juice and pepper.

3. Cut the fish from either side of the central bone and serve with the spinach and the cooking juices from the roasting tin poured over.

Per portion: 298 kcal, 13g fat, 1.4g sat fat, 0.20g sodium, 16g carbohydrate

Trout Saltimbocca

This classic Italian recipe usually uses veal but it's delicious with trout too. Serve with couscous and courgettes, new potatoes or warm cannellini beans and broccoli.

SERVES 4

4 trout fillets, about 125g each, skinned
12 large sage leaves
4 slices Parma ham
1 teaspoon unsalted butter
juice of ½ lemon
freshly ground black pepper

1. Preheat the oven to 190°C/375°F/gas mark 5.

2. Rinse the trout fillets and pat dry with kitchen paper. Season with pepper and lay two sage leaves on one side of each fillet. Fold over then wrap in a slice of Parma ham. Secure with cocktail sticks.

3. Set the fish in a small ovenproof baking dish and cook, covered, for 15 minutes.

4. Heat the butter in a small non-stick frying pan. Finely shred the remaining sage leaves and stir into the butter. Cook until lightly crisp then pour in the cooking juices from the trout and add lemon juice to taste. Spoon over the fish and serve at once.

Per portion: 191 kcal, 8g fat, 1.5g sat fat, 0.41g sodium, 1g carbohydrate

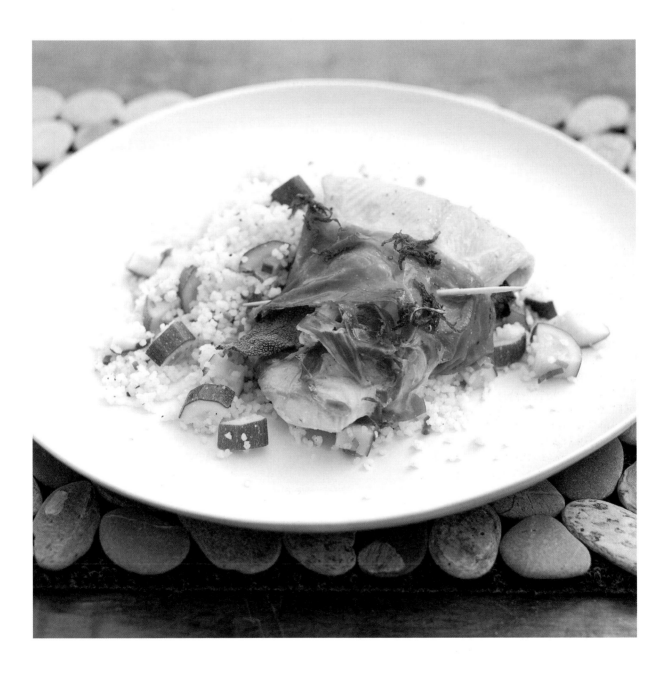

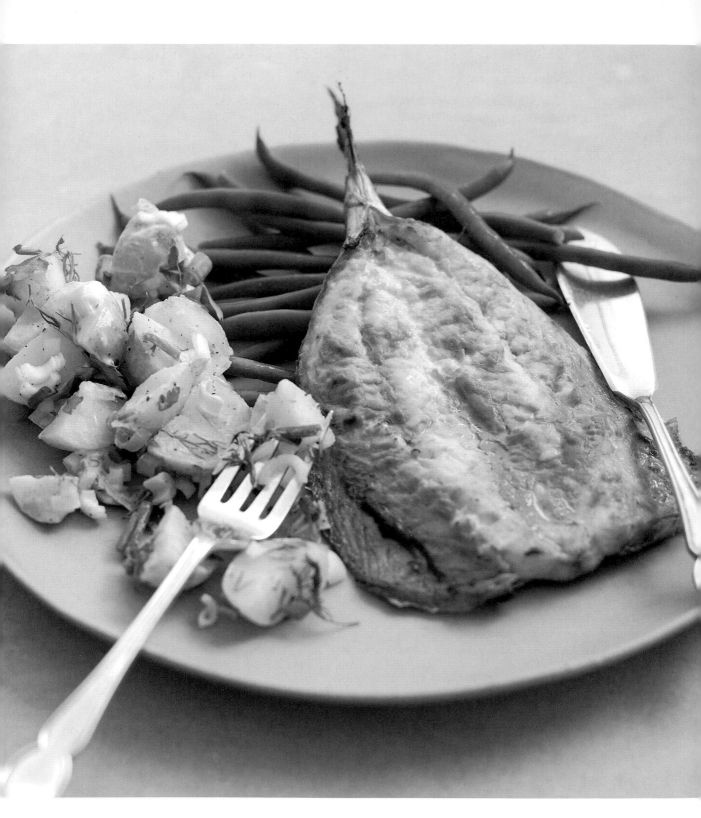

Dijon Mackerel with Scandinavian Potato Salad

One of the simplest yet so tasty ways to prepare mackerel. Ask the fishmonger to clean and fillet the mackerel for you.

SERVES 4

4 mackerel, about 250g each, filleted weight
4 teaspoons Dijon mustard
green beans, to serve

SALAD
400g new potatoes
2 dill pickle cucumbers, chopped
4 spring onions, chopped
1 tablespoon freshly chopped dill
1 tablespoon freshly snipped chives
1 tablespoon freshly chopped parsley
1 tablespoon lemon juice
2 tablespoons reduced-fat fromage frais
freshly ground black pepper

1. For the salad, steam the potatoes until tender – about 20 minutes. Roughly chop, mix with the remaining ingredients and season with pepper to taste.

2. Preheat the grill to high. Wash the mackerel and pat dry on kitchen paper, ensuring that all the black skin from the gut has been removed. Lay the fillets skin-side down and spread the flesh with mustard.

3. Grill the mackerel for about 5 minutes until the flesh is no longer translucent. Serve at once with the potato salad and some green beans.

Per portion: 371 kcal, 21g fat, 4.3g sat fat, 0.34g sodium, 18g carbohydrate

Poached Skate with a Fresh Mediterranean Sauce

Another very easy dish to cook that is also full of flavour. Skate wing fillet is long and wide, but quite meaty, but some species of skate, especially the common skate, are in short supply, so try to choose fish from sustainable sources.

SERVES 2

2 skate wings, about 350g each, cut in half
     if preferred
½ lemon, thinly sliced
1 small onion, peeled and thinly sliced
2 bay leaves
½ teaspoon peppercorns

SAUCE
1 teaspoon coriander seeds
juice of ½ lemon
25g black olives, pitted and chopped
2 spring onions, finely chopped
2 tomatoes, finely chopped
8 large basil leaves, torn in small pieces
freshly ground black pepper

1. Wash the skate pieces and put them in a large wide shallow saucepan with all the flavouring ingredients. Just cover with cold water. Bring to a simmer then cover and simmer very gently for 8–10 minutes until no longer translucent. Drain thoroughly.

2. Meanwhile, toast the coriander seeds in a small dry frying pan over a medium heat until fragrant. Crush with a mortar and pestle and combine with the remaining sauce ingredients. Season with pepper and spoon over the fish. Serve at once with steamed new potatoes and stir-fried courgettes.

Per portion: 261 kcal, 3g fat, 0.3g sat fat, 0.71g sodium, 4g carbohydrate

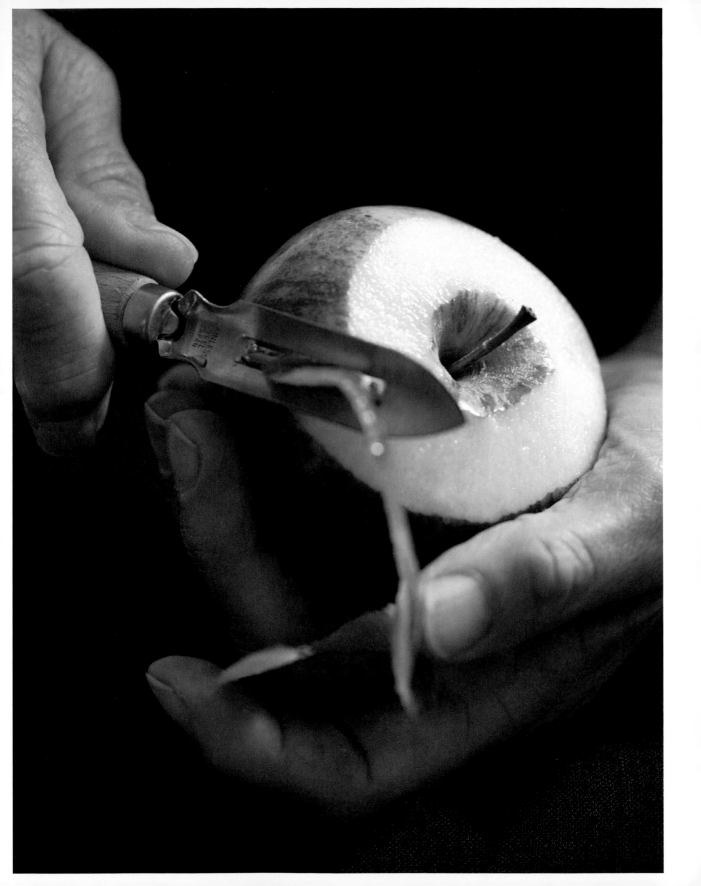

Fruit

About fruit

Fruits in general are low-calorie and low-fat foods and provide vitamin C and other antioxidants and dietary fibre. They should be part of your 'five a day' allowance (page 76). You need to eat at least 400g of fruit and vegetables combined. If there is one fruit that you do not like in a recipe, you can always substitute another, for example replacing plums in a crumble with rhubarb or apple.

Buying frozen fruit enables you to enjoy fruit all year round. You can also freeze fruit to take advantage of surpluses from the garden or bargains on the market stalls. You need to freeze your crop quickly though, as nutrients are lost rapidly after picking.

Dried fruits are another option. Try dried cranberries as a snack as well as the more familiar sultanas and raisins. Remember though that when fruit is dried the water is lost as well as some of the vitamins such as vitamin C. The sugar content is left however so in comparing the weight of dried fruit versus fresh fruit, the dried will have a greater concentration of sugar. So try not to each too much dried fruit at a time – a maximum of about 25g should be your aim. Dried dates have a GI greater than that of glucose itself so keep them for the occasional treat.

If you choose tinned fruits, use those tinned in fruit juice or water, as they are lower in calories than fruits in syrup.

Fruit juice also counts in your 'five a day' but when buying, try to select juices without added sugar and vary the type you choose. Often, combining two different juices – apple and pear for instance – can give a novel flavour. You should also use fruit juice instead of concentrated squashes and cordials.

Smoothies offer all of the goodness of fruit as they also include the fibre, so they make a useful alternative to a piece of fruit. Many people find they make a quick, revitalising breakfast.

Low GI and GL fruits

Rhubarb is wonderfully low in calories, GI and GL so is useful in a wide range of desserts.

Apples, bananas, pears, cherries, grapefruit, strawberries, kiwi, oranges, peaches, plums, gooseberries, cranberries, strawberries, blackberries, loganberries, blueberries and raspberries all have a low GI and can be enjoyed as snacks or as part of dishes.

Other fruits

Watermelon and pineapple have a higher GI but because they are eaten in relatively small amounts (100g) their GL is not particularly high.

What constitutes a portion of fruit

A medium apple, peach, banana or pear

Half a large fruit such as a grapefruit

Two plums

A slice of melon, mango, or pineapple

A teacup or handful of berries or grapes

Three tablespoons of tinned or stewed fruit

Dried fruit – about the same amount as if the fruit were fresh e.g. 3 apricots or 2 figs

A small glass or carton of fruit juice – this only counts as one portion, no matter how much you drink, as the fibre is removed during the processing.

Banana, Raspberry and Crunchy Oat Yogurt Fool

A simple dessert and any leftovers will be great for breakfast!

SERVES 4

25g oat flakes or rye flakes
2 tablespoons raw cane demerara sugar
500g 0.1% fat natural yogurt
½ teaspoon natural vanilla extract
2 bananas, peeled and roughly mashed
125g raspberries, fresh or frozen

1. Put the oat flakes and sugar in a small non-stick frying pan and cook, stirring, over a medium heat until the flakes are lightly toasted and the sugar has caramelised. Leave to cool then break into small clusters.

2. Combine all the remaining ingredients and just before serving, stir in the caramelised oat flakes. Serve at once.

Per portion: 188 kcal, 2g fat, 1.0g sat fat, 0.08g sodium, 37g carbohydrate

Grilled Figs with Pancetta

A delicious starter or snack to serve on a slice of toast or with a green salad garnish.

SERVES 2

4 large ripe figs
freshly ground black pepper
8 slices pancetta
8 small sprigs of fresh thyme

1. Preheat the grill to high.

2. Wash and dry the figs, cut in half and season with pepper. Wrap each fig half in a slice of pancetta, tucking in a thyme sprig as you go. Secure with cocktail sticks.

3. Grill for 3–4 minutes on each side until the pancetta is crispy. Serve at once.

Per portion: 328 kcal, 10g fat, 0g sat fat, 0.61g sodium, 54g carbohydrate

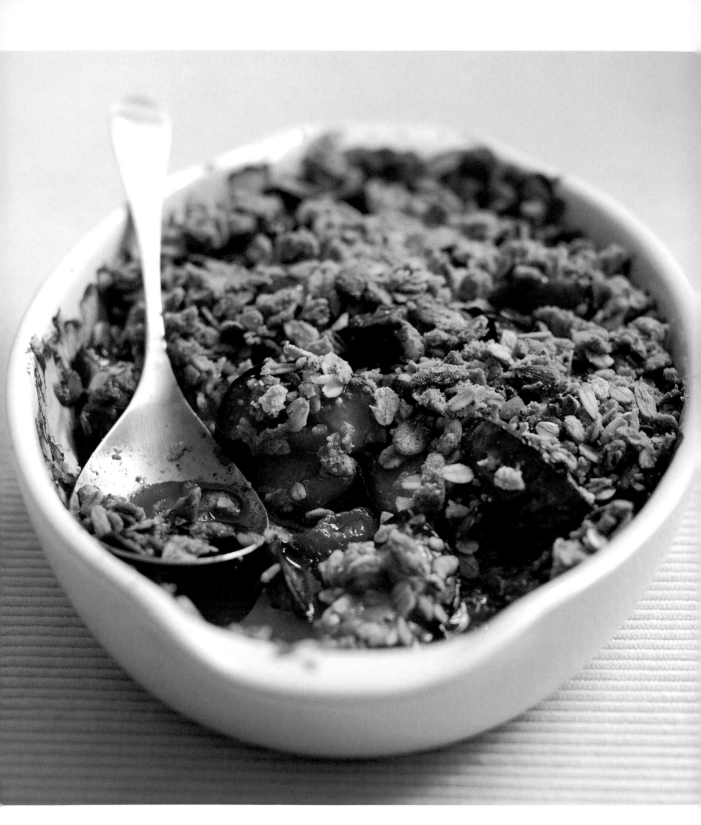

Plum Oat Crumble

Greengages or apricots may be used as an alternative to red plums.

SERVES 4–6

750g red plums, quartered and stoned
25g raw cane brown sugar
50g whole, rolled porridge oats
25g wholemeal flour with malted wheatgrains
25g pumpkin seeds (or sunflower seeds)
½ teaspoon ground cinnamon
½ teaspoon ground ginger
25g unsalted butter, softened

1. Preheat the oven to 190°C/375°F/gas mark 5. Place the plum quarters in a shallow gratin dish and, only if they are firm, sprinkle with 3 tablespoons water.

2. Mix together the sugar, oats, flour, seeds and spices and rub in the butter. Sprinkle over the plums and bake for 35–45 minutes until the plums are tender.

3. Serve with natural yogurt or vanilla ice cream.

Per portion: 248 kcal, 9g fat, 3.7g sat fat, 0.01g sodium, 39g carbohydrate

Baked Breakfast Fruits

Great with a dollop of natural yogurt.

SERVES 8

125g small stoned prunes
125g small dried apricots or figs
125g dried apple rings
75g raisins
3 bananas, peeled and thickly sliced
4 cardamom pods, split
2 tablespoons clear honey
finely grated zest of 1 orange and juice of
    2 oranges
finely grated zest of ½ lemon

1. Place the prunes, apricots and apple rings in a bowl and cover with boiling water from the kettle. Cover and leave to soak overnight.

2. The following day, preheat the oven to 180°C/350°F/gas mark 4. Drain the fruits well and transfer to a large baking dish. Add the raisins, banana slices and cardamom pods.

3. Combine the honey, citrus fruit zest and 125ml water and pour over the fruits. Mix together.

4. Bake for 35 minutes then stir in the orange juice. Serve warm.

Per portion: 167 kcal, 0.4g fat, 0.1g sat fat, 0.02g sodium, 41g carbohydrate

Pears, Prunes, Oranges and Pecans in Spiced Port Wine

A perfect dessert for an autumn or winter supper.

SERVES 4–6

5 tablespoons ruby port
finely grated zest and juice of 1 orange
juice of 1 small lemon
2 tablespoons redcurrant jelly
2 bay leaves
½ teaspoon ground cinnamon
½ teaspoon ground nutmeg
4 medium ripe pears, quartered and cored –
   do not peel
8 large ready-to-eat prunes
2 large oranges
12 pecan halves

1. Pour the port into a measuring jug and make up to 300ml with water. Pour into a large saucepan and add the next six ingredients. Bring to a simmer then add the pear quarters, cover and simmer for about 20 minutes until almost tender.

2. Add the prunes and boil rapidly for 5 minutes to reduce the liquid. Leave to cool.

3. Peel the oranges with a small serrated knife to remove all the white pith, then cut in thin slices. Stir into the pear mixture together with the pecans.

4. Serve on its own or with natural yogurt.

Per portion: 281 kcal, 7g fat, 0.6g sat fat, 0.02g sodium, 49g carbohydrate

Luxury Fruit Salad

A refreshing fruit salad with a touch of the Caribbean, this is perfect for a party – and the leftovers are delicious for breakfast. Dried coconut slices are available from good health food shops. Fresh coconut (for grating) can be found in most supermarkets. Please don't be tempted to use desiccated coconut in this recipe!

SERVES 8

finely grated zest and juice of 2 limes
2 tablespoons golden caster sugar
150ml orange juice (use blood orange juice if
   available)
2 passion fruit, halved, seeds and pulp removed
1 mango, peeled
1 papaya, peeled and seeds removed
½ medium pineapple, peeled
125g watermelon flesh
½ medium sweet melon, peeled and seeds
   removed
75g shredded fresh coconut or dried coconut
   slices (optional)

1. Combine the lime zest and juice, sugar, orange juice and passion fruit seeds and pulp in a large bowl.

2. Cut all the remaining fruit in bite-sized pieces and add to the bowl. Mix well and serve at once or cover and chill in the fridge until required.

Per portion: 91 kcal, 0g fat, 0g sat fat, 0.04g sodium, 22g carbohydrate

Baked Peaches with Brown Sugar and Almonds

This is best made when good-quality ripe peaches are available in the shops.

SERVES 4

4 tablespoons flaked almonds
4 large ripe peaches, halved and stoned
2 tablespoons raw cane soft brown sugar
1 teaspoon ground ginger
150ml freshly squeezed orange juice
low-fat natural yogurt, to serve

1. Preheat the oven to 190°C/375°F/gas mark 5. Spread the almonds on a baking sheet and toast for about 10 minutes until golden.

2. Arrange the peach halves cut side up in a gratin dish. Mix together the toasted almonds, sugar and ginger and sprinkle into the centre of each peach half.

3. Pour the orange juice around the fruit and bake, uncovered, for about 25 minutes until tender.

4. Serve on its own or with natural yogurt

Per portion: 198 kcal, 9g fat, 0.7g sat fat, 0.01g sodium, 26g carbohydrate

Peach and Blueberry Gratin

A very simple dessert using tinned peaches in fruit juice. You can substitute ripe fresh peaches when in season.

SERVES 4

410g tinned peach halves in fruit juice
   (or 3 large ripe peaches)
175g blueberries
300g 0% fat Greek yogurt
50g amaretti or ratafia biscuits, roughly crumbled
1 teaspoon ground cinnamon

1. Preheat the grill to medium-high. Drain the peaches and reserve 2 tablespoons juice. Cut each peach half into four slices and divide them between 4 ramekin dishes. Add the blueberries.

2. Spread the yogurt over the top. Mix the crumbled biscuits with the cinnamon and moisten with the reserved fruit juice. Scatter over the yogurt and grill for 2–3 minutes until lightly caramelised. Serve at once.

Per portion: 135 kcal, 0g fat, 0g sat fat, 0.01g sodium, 13g carbohydrate

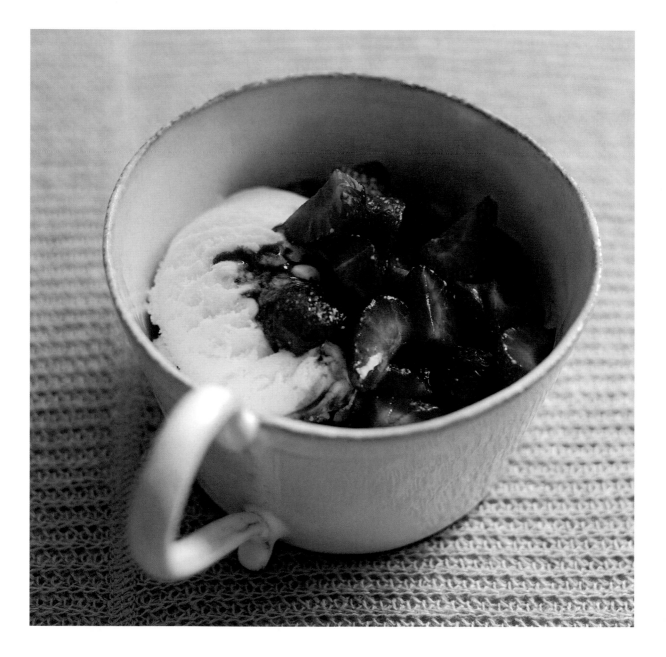

Balsamic Strawberries with Vanilla Ice Cream

Simple yet no less effective for that! Make sure you buy an aged balsamic vinegar (not cheap but worth every penny) so that the juices produced by the strawberries will have a delicious, slightly fruity tang rather than being astringent, which will happen if you use a cheap vinegar.

SERVES 4

1 x 454g punnet ripe strawberries
2 tablespoons golden icing sugar
2 teaspoons aged balsamic vinegar
    (or lemon juice or ruby port)
4 scoops vanilla ice cream
    (or vanilla ice non-dairy dessert)

1. Wash the strawberries then pat dry on kitchen paper. Remove the hulls and cut in quarters.

2. Sprinkle with the icing sugar and vinegar and leave for up to 1 hour at room temperature to macerate.

3. Serve with a scoop of vanilla ice cream.

Per portion: 176 kcal, 5g fat, 3.7g sat fat, 0.04g sodium, 29g carbohydrate

A Fruit Salad of Mango, Strawberries and Blueberries with Fresh Lime

The lime produces a refreshing, clean-tasting syrup to enhance the fruit flavours. Perfect for breakfast.

SERVES 4–6

2 large ripe mangoes
175g small ripe strawberries, washed, hulled
    and halved
175g blueberries
25g golden caster sugar
finely grated zest and juice of 2 small limes

1. Peel and slice the mangoes, discarding the stones, and combine with the berries.

2. Sprinkle with the sugar, lime zest and juice and leave to macerate for up to 1 hour to release the juices.

Per portion: 92 kcal, 0.4g fat, 0.1g sat fat, 0.01g sodium, 23g carbohydrate

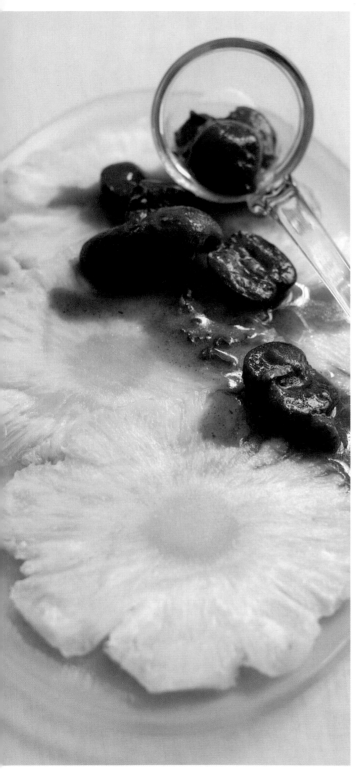

Carpaccio of Pineapple with Spiced Cherries

'Carpaccio' usually means very thin slices of raw beef but in this recipe it simply refers to the wafer-thin slices of pineapple that are used.

SERVES 4

½ very large sweet ripe pineapple

SPICED CHERRIES
250g fresh cherries, stoned and halved
15g unsalted butter
15g golden caster sugar
large pinch of ground cinnamon
large pinch of ground nutmeg
1 teaspoon arrowroot mixed with 1 tablespoon
    cold water
½ tablespoon freshly chopped mint

1. Place the cherries, butter, sugar and spices in a saucepan with 100ml water and bring to a simmer. Simmer very gently, uncovered, for 5 minutes then stir in the arrowroot and cook, stirring, until lightly thickened. Remove from the heat and add the mint. Leave to cool.

2. Peel the pineapple, removing all the 'eyes', and using a large serrated knife, cut in wafer-thin slices. Arrange the slices in a thin layer on 4 dinner plates. Spoon some cherries onto the centre of each plate and serve.

Per portion: 100 kcal, 3g fat, 2.0g sat fat, 0g sodium, 18g carbohydrate

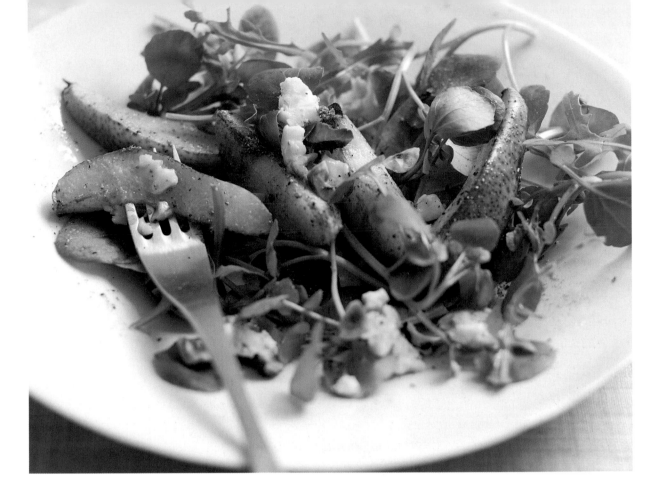

Pan-Fried Pear Salad with Hazelnuts and Blue Cheese

A little blue cheese goes a long way because of its strong flavour.

SERVES 2

2 ripe pears
1 teaspoon unsalted butter
1 teaspoon olive oil
¼ teaspoon ground coriander
freshly ground black pepper
100g mixed rocket, watercress and
   baby spinach leaves
25g blue cheese such as Gorgonzola, Dolcelatte
   or Saint Agur, crumbled
1 tablespoon hazelnuts, roasted and
   roughly chopped
1 tablespoon lemon juice

1. Quarter and core the pears then cut each quarter in half. Heat the butter and oil in a large non-stick frying pan, add the pears and cook for about 3 minutes on each side until golden. Season with the ground coriander and pepper.

2. Lightly toss with all the remaining ingredients and serve at once.

**Per portion: 195 kcal, 13g fat, 1.9g sat fat,
0.15g sodium, 17g carbohydrate**

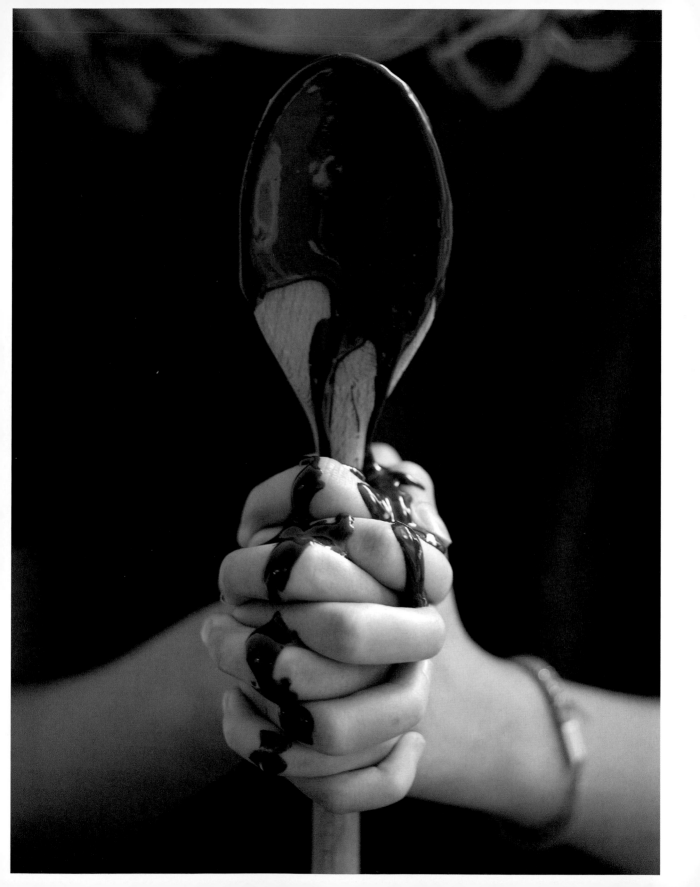

Sweet treats

About sweet treats

Most people like sweet-tasting foods. The sweetness comes from the various sugars used but these are a form of carbohydrate, which adds to the calorie content. In addition, sugars do not contain any nutrients, which is why they are often referred to as 'empty calories'. The frequent consumption of excessive amounts of sugar are also associated with tooth decay. The secret, then, is to make sure that you do not eat too many sweet foods and that you eat them at meal times and in recipes that include low GI foods. Regard them as treats that add variety to your diet.

The recipes in this book use small amounts of sugar for sweetness. Honey, golden syrup, molasses, corn syrup, malt extract and treacle contain sugars in thick, sticky solutions and can also be used to add flavour. Try using different sugars and syrups for a change.

Glucose

Glucose is a simple sugar and has a GI of 100, so should be avoided. It is not used as an ingredient in home cooking except sometimes in cake icings. If you check packets of ready-made cakes and confectionery, you will find that glucose syrup and corn syrup are used. Glucose is also a major ingredient in some sports drinks and sweetened drinks.

Sucrose

Sucrose, or table sugar, has a medium GI of 68 and as it is pure carbohydrate a 100g will provide a high GL. However as only small amounts need to be used in recipes with other low GL ingredients, it can be used for flavour.

Fructose

This is another simple sugar like glucose but the body handles it in a different way, which is why it has a low GI of only 19. It is the sugar found particularly in fruits and, like glucose and sucrose, it is a carbohydrate.

Some people like to use it in cooking instead of sucrose but it can upset the digestion if eaten in excess.

Using sugars

It is sensible to try to limit the amount of sugar you eat both to save calories and for dental health. So try to avoid adding sugar to tea, coffee and cereals but use it where it makes a contribution to the texture and flavour of a recipe or where it will help you to enjoy your food. For example, eat your porridge with a spoonful of syrup and your grain toast with jam instead of butter or spread.

It is obviously better to buy tinned fruit and drinks that do not contain added sugar (see page 130). Similarly, avoid sweetened breakfast cereals and use fruit to add sweetness instead. Try not to add sugar to tea and coffee – it is often best to cut down gradually over several weeks.

Hazelnut Meringues

These will keep in an airtight container in a cool dry place for up to 1 month. When ready to serve, fill each one with 2 tablespoons low-fat fromage frais or natural yogurt and 50g fresh berries.

MAKES 12

50g hazelnuts
4 egg whites
pinch of cream of tartar
225g golden caster sugar

1. Preheat the oven to 180°C/350°F/gas mark 4. Spread the hazelnuts on a baking sheet and roast for 15–20 minutes until golden. Allow to cool slightly, then whizz in a food-processor until quite finely chopped or chop by hand.

2. Reduce the oven temperature to 130°C/275°F/ gas mark 1. Line 1–2 baking trays with non-stick baking parchment or non-stick baking plastic.

3. Whisk the egg whites with the cream of tartar until stiff, then whisk in the sugar, a tablespoonful at a time, until the mixture is stiff once more. When you lift the whisks out of the mixture it should hold in firm peaks.

4. Fold in the roasted hazelnuts then spoon 12 rough ovals of the mixture, spaced well apart, onto the prepared baking tray(s) and make a small hollow in each. Bake for 1¼–1½ hours until crisp and dry. Leave to cool then store in an air-tight container (see above).

Per meringue: 105 kcal, 3g fat, 0.2g sat fat, 0.02g sodium, 20g carbohydrate

Lemon Blancmanges with Honeyed Blackberries

A recipe from my childhood that deserves a comeback!

SERVES 4

600ml semi-skimmed milk
pared zest of 2 lemons and juice of 1 lemon
40g cornflour
50g golden caster sugar
150g blackberries, fresh or frozen (or frozen fruits of the forest)
1 tablespoon clear honey
4 small sprigs of lemon balm, to decorate (optional)

1. Put three-quarters of the milk in a saucepan with the pared lemon zest. Bring just to a simmer then turn off the heat and leave to infuse for 15 minutes. Strain to remove the zest, return to the pan and keep warm.

2. Mix the cornflour and sugar to a paste with the rest of the milk in a bowl. Pour the lemon-infused milk over the cornflour mixture and mix well. Return to the pan and cook, stirring, until thickened. Simmer very gently for at least 5 minutes, stirring frequently, until the cornflour is thoroughly cooked and no longer tastes powdery.

3. Remove from the heat and slowly beat in the lemon juice. Divide between 4 wetted 150ml individual moulds. Leave to cool then cover and chill in the fridge for at least 3–4 hours until set firm.

4. Warm the berries with the honey and 1 tablespoon water. Unmould the blancmanges onto 4 plates and spoon a few berries onto each plate. Decorate with sprigs of lemon balm.

Per blancmange: 178 kcal, 3g fat, 1.6g sat fat, 0.07g sodium, 35g carbohydrate

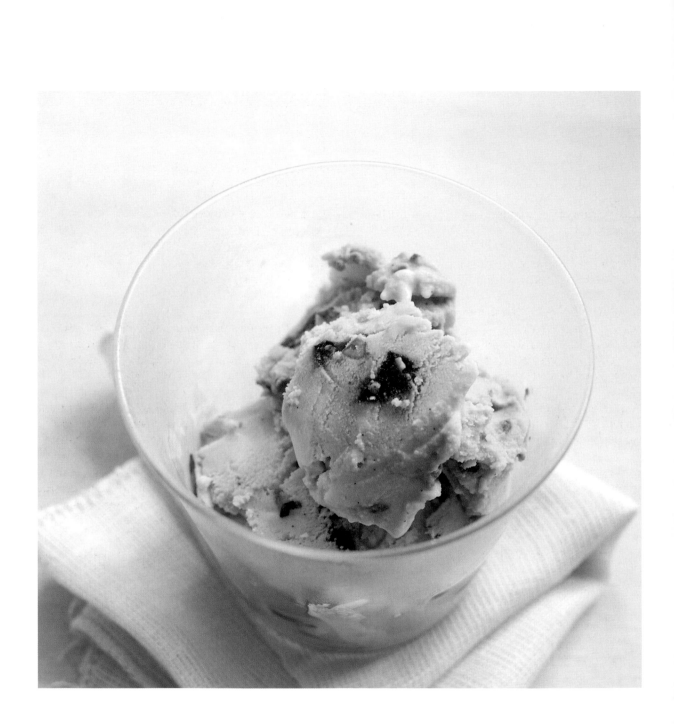

Cherry and Toasted Pine Nut Frozen Yogurt

Ideally you need an ice-cream machine to obtain a wonderfully smooth texture. If you do not have one, freeze the mixture in a rigid container then beat well before adding the flavouring ingredients.

SERVES 4

450g 3% fat (or whole-fat) Greek-style yogurt
2 tablespoons clear honey
½ vanilla pod
4 tablespoons semi-skimmed milk
15g pine nuts
100g fresh cherries, stoned and halved

1. Combine the yogurt, honey, seeds scraped from the vanilla pod and the milk, and transfer to an ice-cream machine (see above). Churn for 10–15 minutes until softly whipped and almost frozen.

2. Meanwhile dry-fry the pine nuts in a small non-stick frying pan over a medium heat, stirring until lightly toasted. Leave to cool.

3. Add the nuts and cherries to the yogurt mixture and continue churning for about 5 minutes. Serve straight away or transfer to a rigid container and store in the freezer. Allow to soften slightly at room temperature before serving with Cats' Tongues (see opposite).

Per portion: 227 kcal, 14g fat, 7.9g sat fat, 0.08g sodium, 18g carbohydrate

Cats' Tongues

Also known as *langues de chat*, these lovely, light biscuits are delicious by themselves or with tea, coffee, frozen yogurt and ice cream. Also another great use for the non-stick baking plastic.

MAKES 40

50g unsalted butter
50g golden caster sugar
50g plain white flour
1 teaspoon natural vanilla extract
2 egg whites

1. Preheat the oven to 220°C/425°F/gas mark 7. Line 2 baking trays with non-stick baking plastic or non-stick baking parchment.

2. Cream the butter and sugar until pale and fluffy then beat in the flour followed by the vanilla extract. Beat in the egg white a little at a time to give a smooth, thick mixture.

3. Use the mixture to fill a piping bag fitted with a 6mm nozzle. Pipe 40 short lengths (7.5–9 cm) of mixture, spaced well apart, on the baking trays.

4. Bake for 8–10 minutes until tinged golden at the edges. Cool slightly on the trays then transfer to a wire rack until completely cold and crisp. Store in an airtight container.

Per biscuit: 19 kcal, 1g fat, 0.7g sat fat, 0g sodium, 2g carbohydrate

Chocolate Semi-Freddo

This chocolate terrine can be sliced straight from the freezer – you should then allow about 15 minutes for each slice to 'come to' before serving. Delicious with a few raspberries.

SERVES 10–12

100g ready-to-eat dried figs, chopped
1 tablespoon candied peel
1 tablespoon dried cranberries
1 tablespoon dried cherries
1 tablespoon dried blueberries
1 apple-flavoured green tea bag
175g good-quality dark chocolate, minimum
    70% cocoa solids, chopped
25g golden caster sugar
2 eggs, separated
25g cocoa powder, sifted
300g 0% fat Greek yogurt
fresh raspberries, to serve

1. Place the dried fruits in a small bowl with the tea bag and cover with 100ml boiling water. Cover and leave to soak overnight. The following day, squeeze out the teabag and discard.

2. Line a 900g loaf tin or terrine with a double thickness of cling film so that it overlaps the edges enough to fold back over the top.

3. Melt the chocolate either in the microwave or over a saucepan of simmering water. Whisk together the sugar, egg yolks and cocoa powder then fold in the yogurt, melted chocolate and finally the macerated fruit together with any liquid.

4. Whisk the egg whites until soft peaks form and fold through the chocolate mixture. Transfer to the tin, level the surface and freeze overnight. Serve, cut in slices, with a few berries to decorate.

Per portion: 171 kcal, 7g fat, 3.6g sat fat, 0.05g sodium, 22g carbohydrate

Hot Chocolate Soufflés

These impressive soufflés can be made in individual ramekins or coffee cups.

SERVES 6

3 tablespoons cornflour
1 tablespoon cocoa powder
250ml semi-skimmed milk
50g good-quality dark chocolate, minimum
    70% cocoa solids, chopped
4 eggs, separated
3 tablespoons golden caster sugar
golden icing sugar, to dust
fresh berries, to serve (optional)

SAUCE
50g good-quality chocolate, minimum
    70% cocoa solids, chopped
1 tablespoon cocoa powder
1 tablespoon golden caster sugar
200ml semi-skimmed milk

1. Lightly butter six individual ramekin dishes or cups (120ml capacity) then sprinkle the insides with a little caster sugar and shake off the excess. Chill until required. Preheat the oven to 190°C/375°F/gas mark 5 and put a baking tray in the oven to heat.

2. Mix the cornflour and cocoa powder to a smooth paste in a bowl with some of the milk. Warm the rest of the milk in a pan with the chocolate until melted, then pour onto the cornflour and mix until smooth. Return to the pan and simmer, stirring all the time, until smooth and thickened. Cook very gently for 5 minutes, stirring frequently, then remove from the heat and beat in the egg yolks one at a time.

3. Whisk the egg whites in a clean bowl until stiff then whisk in the golden caster sugar, a tablespoon at a time. Fold a little of the egg-white mixture into the chocolate mixture then fold that through the egg whites until evenly combined.

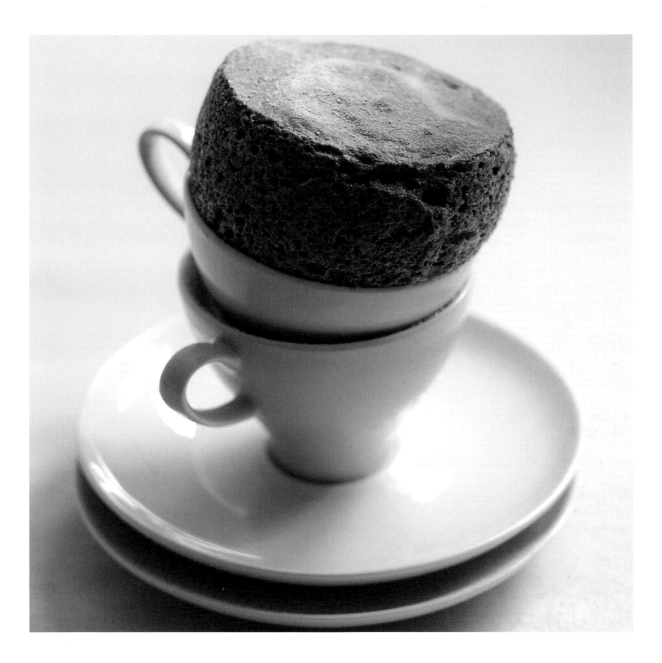

4. Divide between the prepared ramekins then run your finger between the inside edge of the ramekin and the mixture to make a small groove (see page 95). Set the ramekins on the baking tray and cook towards the top of the oven for 10–12 minutes until well risen and just wobbly when lightly moved.

5. Meanwhile, warm all the sauce ingredients in a pan until the chocolate is melted, then simmer gently for 5 minutes, whisking occasionally. Dust the soufflés with icing sugar and serve at once with the chocolate sauce and berries, if wished.

Per portion: 288 kcal, 11g fat, 5.2g sat fat, 0.13g sodium, 42g carbohydrate

Spiced Sponge Roll with Berries

This is a great gluten-free roll. It's perfect with a cup of tea or as a dessert with a dollop of low-fat natural yogurt or low-fat fromage frais. Any leftovers will taste very like Summer Pudding the next day!

SERVES 8

4 eggs, separated
100g golden caster sugar
3 tablespoons arrowroot
3 tablespoons cornflour
1 teaspoon ground cinnamon
1 teaspoon ground ginger
1 teaspoon ground mixed spice
1 tablespoon golden syrup or honey
350g assorted fresh berries, such as raspberries, blackberries, blueberries, chopped strawberries
golden icing sugar, to dust

1. Preheat the oven to 190°C/375°F/gas mark 5. Line a 35cm x 25cm Swiss roll tin with non-stick baking parchment.

2. Whisk the egg whites until stiff then whisk in half the sugar, a spoonful at a time, until thick and glossy. Sift the remaining sugar with the rest of the dry ingredients and whisk into the egg whites, a spoonful at a time. Fold in the egg yolks and golden syrup just until evenly mixed.

3. Spread the mixture in the prepared tin and level the surface. Bake for 10 minutes until risen and golden and just firm to the touch.

4. Lay a sheet of non-stick baking parchment the same size as the tin on a work surface and sprinkle liberally with icing sugar. Turn the sponge out onto the sugared paper.

5. Spread the fruit evenly over the sponge leaving a 3cm gap at each of the short ends. Make an indentation along the length of one short end (to help with the rolling)and start rolling up the sponge, enclosing the fruit as you go and using the paper to guide you.

6. As soon as the sponge is rolled, remove the paper. Dust the surface of the roll with icing sugar. Serve fresh on the day of making.

Per portion: 162 kcal, 3g fat, 1.0g sat fat, 0.05g sodium, 31g carbohydrate

Plum Jam

There's nothing quite like home-made jam and this version is easy to make and foolproof. Choose from a variety of plums or greengages.

MAKES ABOUT 1.7KG

2kg plums, halved, stoned and roughly chopped
1kg raw cane granulated or caster sugar

1. Put the plums and sugar in a stainless-steel preserving pan. Stir well, cover and leave for at least 4 hours, until the juices run.

2. Bring slowly to a simmer, stirring frequently, until the sugar dissolves, then bring to the boil. Boil gently for 1½ hours until thickened, stirring frequently, so that it does not stick to the bottom of the pan: there is no need to test it with a thermometer.

3. About 15 minutes before the jam is ready, preheat the oven to 180°C/350°F/gas mark 4. Put several clean jam jars in the oven to warm for 10 minutes. When the jam is ready, transfer to the jars, filling them to the top. Cover each with a waxed paper disc and leave to cool. Cover and label, then store in a cool place.

Per tablespoon (about 44g): 69 kcal, 0g fat, 0g sat fat, 0g sodium, 18g carbohydrate

Greek Cherry Glyko

'Glyko' translates as anything sweet and in traditional Greek households a spoonful or two of home-made sweet glyko is usually presented to visiting women while the men get an ouzo or whisky! I think it's better spread on bread or stirred into Greek yogurt than eaten from a spoon.

If you prefer a firmer set then replace the sugar with 'jam sugar' which has added pectin.

MAKES ABOUT 1.2KG

1.25kg cherries, stoned
250ml fresh lemon juice
750g raw cane granulated or caster sugar

1. Put all the ingredients in a stainless-steel preserving pan. Stir well, cover and leave for at least 4 hours, until the juices run.

2. Bring slowly to a simmer, stirring frequently, until the sugar dissolves, then bring to the boil.

3. Boil gently for about 45 minutes , stirring frequently, until the sugar thermometer reaches 105°C/220°F. Remove from the heat and leave to settle for 15 minutes.

4. Meanwhile, preheat the oven to 180°C/350°F/gas mark 4. Put several clean jam jars in the oven to warm for 10 minutes. When the jam is ready, transfer to the jars, filling them to the top. Cover each with a waxed paper disc and leave to cool. Cover and label, then store in a cool place.

VARIATION
Stir in 100g roasted, chopped almonds once the jam has reached 105°C/220°F.

Per tablespoon (about 47g): 74 kcal, 0g fat, 0g sat fat, 0g sodium, 20g carbohydrate

Hot Mochas

A great nightcap or mid-morning treat!

MAKES 2

1 tablespoon cocoa powder
1 tablespoon golden caster sugar
300ml semi-skimmed milk
25g good-quality chocolate, minimum 70%
   cocoa solids, chopped
300ml freshly brewed strong coffee

1. In a small saucepan, mix the cocoa powder and sugar to a paste with some of the milk then add the rest of the milk and the chocolate and bring to a simmer, whisking all the time until the chocolate has melted.

2. Stir in the coffee and warm to the required temperature. Serve at once.

Per portion: 186 kcal, 7g fat, 4.3g sat fat, 0.11g sodium, 26g carbohydrate

Almond and Apricot Pavlova Slice

You can make and bake the basic pavlova mixture up to 1 week in advance then store in a cool, dry place until required.

SERVES 8–10

3 tablespoons ground almonds
5 large egg whites
pinch of cream of tartar
250g golden caster sugar
2 teaspoons cornflour
1 teaspoon white wine vinegar
½ teaspoon natural almond extract
25g amaretti biscuits, crushed
125g ready-to-eat dried apricots, diced

FILLING
300g 0% fat Greek yogurt
1 ripe peach, stoned and thinly sliced
1 medium mango, peeled and thinly sliced
1 large orange, segmented and all pith and
   membrane removed

1. Preheat the oven to 180°C/350°F/gas mark 4. Line a shallow 35cm x 25cm baking tray with non-stick baking parchment to come at least 3cm up the sides.

2. In a dry non-stick frying pan, toast the ground almonds over a medium heat, stirring all the time until golden.

3. Whisk the egg whites with the cream of tartar until stiff then whisk in the sugar, a spoonful at a time, until you have one spoonful left. Mix the cornflour into that and whisk into the egg whites until stiff and glossy. Whisk in the vinegar and almond extract and finally fold in the toasted almonds, crushed amaretti and apricots.

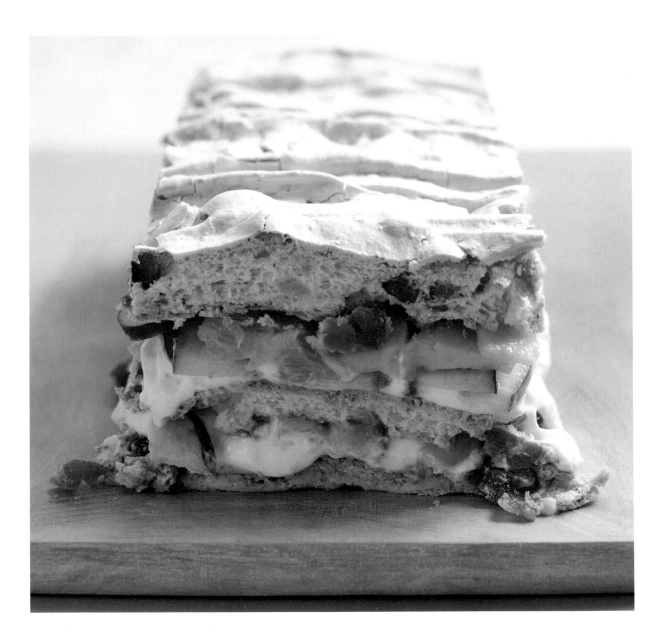

4. Spread the mixture into the prepared baking tray and level the surface. Place in the oven and immediately reduce the temperature to 150°C/300°F/gas mark 2. Cook for 45 minutes until pale golden and crisp on top. Turn off the oven, leave the door ajar and allow to cool.

5. Remove from the tray, trim the edges and cut across the shorter side to make 3 equal pieces. Spread two pieces with yogurt and layer on the fruit. Sandwich together, press down gently, then cut in slices to serve.

Per slice: 284 kcal, 5g fat, 0.4g sat fat, 0.05g sodium, 49g carbohydrate

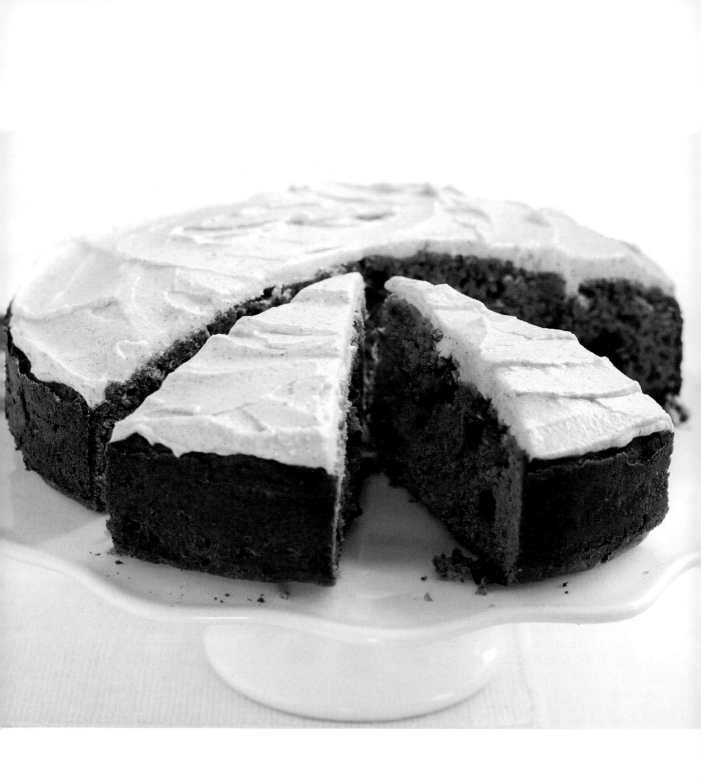

Passion Cake

Store in an airtight container in the fridge, but for no longer than 2–3 days, or freeze.

SERVES 10

3 medium eggs
50g stoned dates
50g unsalted butter, softened
1 ripe pear (about 150g) cored and chopped
150g carrots, coarsely grated
150g gram flour (or gluten-free flour or plain flour)
1 tablespoon wheat-free baking powder
2 teaspoons ground cinnamon
1 teaspoon ground nutmeg
½ teaspoon ground allspice
50g dried berries – a combination of blueberries, cherries and cranberries, or sultanas or raisins
golden icing sugar, to dust (optional)

ICING (OPTIONAL)
125g quark
1 tablespoon golden icing sugar
½ teaspoon ground cinnamon

1. Preheat the oven to 190°C/375°F/gas mark 5. Grease, flour and line the base of a 20cm cake tin with non-stick baking parchment.

2. Put the eggs, dates and butter in a food-processor with 50ml water and whizz until nearly smooth. Add the pear and whizz until smooth. Transfer to a bowl and stir in the carrots.

3. Sift all the dry ingredients together and fold into the fruit mixture. Stir in the berries and transfer to the prepared tin. Level and bake for about 35 minutes until risen and firm. Cool in the tin then transfer to a wire rack until completely cold. Dust with icing sugar, if wished.

4. If desired, beat the icing ingredients together until smooth and spread over the cake.

Per slice: 164 kcal, 6g fat, 3.3g sat fat, 0.21g sodium, 23g carbohydrate

Gingerbread with Pear

Coarse oatmeal produces a very 'nutty' texture so if you prefer, use medium oatmeal instead. The use of fresh pear moistens the cake but also reduces its keeping qualities, so store it in an airtight container in the fridge. You can also replace the fresh pear with 4–6 halves of ready-to-eat dried pear if you wish. Another great stand-by recipe for the freezer.

SERVES 12

150g coarse (or medium) oatmeal
150g strong brown bread flour with wheatgrains
100g raw cane soft brown sugar
2 tablespoons ground ginger
1 teaspoon bicarbonate of soda
100g fruit spread (without added sugar)
2 eggs
2 medium ripe pears, quartered, cored and chopped
4 pieces stem ginger, chopped (optional)

1. Preheat the oven to 180°C/350°F/gas mark 4. Lightly grease and line the base of a 900g loaf tin with non-stick baking parchment.

2. Put all the dry ingredients in a bowl and mix well. Beat the fruit spread with 2 tablespoons boiled water until smooth, then beat in the eggs. Mix into the dry ingredients until well combined.

3. Fold in the pears and ginger, if using, and transfer to the prepared tin. Level the surface and bake in the centre of the oven for about 1 hour until risen and just springy to the touch. It may take an extra 5–10 minutes. If unsure, test with a fine metal skewer which should come out clean when inserted into the centre of the cake.

4. Leave in the tin until cool enough to handle then turn out onto a wire rack. Cover with a clean tea towel and leave until completely cold.

Per slice: 176 kcal, 3g fat, 0.4g sat fat, 0.10g sodium, 36g carbohydrate

Ricotta Fruit Cake

This can be served warm as a dessert or cold as a cake with coffee or tea. It will keep in an airtight container in the fridge for 2–3 days.

SERVES 10

125g unsalted butter, softened
75g golden caster sugar
4 eggs, separated plus 1 egg white
finely grated zest of 1 orange and 1 large lemon
100g mixed dried fruits, such as whole cranberries, whole cherries, whole blueberries and chopped ready-to-eat dried apricots
50g roasted hazelnuts, roughly chopped
150g ricotta
40g strong white bread flour with kibbled grains of wheat and rye
icing sugar, to dust (optional)

1. Preheat the oven to 180°C/350°F/gas mark 4. Butter and line the base of a 19–20cm spring-release tin with non-stick baking parchment. Cream the butter and sugar until pale and fluffy. Add the egg yolks one by one, beating well between each addition. In a separate bowl, fold the zests, fruit and nuts into the ricotta. Fold the butter and egg mix into the ricotta and fruit. Finally fold in the flour until evenly combined.

2. Whisk the egg whites to soft peaks. Fold one large spoonful of egg white into the ricotta mix, then carefully fold in the remainder, ensuring that you do not lose too much of the air. Transfer the mixture to the prepared tin, level the surface and cook for 40–45 minutes or until the tip of a knife or a fine metal skewer inserted into the centre comes out clean.

3. Allow to cool in the tin then transfer to a wire rack. Serve warm or cold, dusted with icing sugar, if wished.

Per slice: 245 kcal, 18g fat, 8.5g sat fat, 0.06g sodium, 16g carbohydrate

Sparkling Elderflower Jellies

An elegant dessert – you can add a touch of glamour by using Champagne or sparking white wine, if you like.

MAKES 4

4 leaves gelatine
100ml elderflower cordial
500ml sparkling mineral water (or Champagne or sparkling white wine)
6 tablespoons fresh raspberries
4 tablespoons fresh blueberries

1. Soak the gelatine in cold water for 10 minutes. Drain and squeeze out the excess water. Pour 4 tablespoons boiling water into a bowl and add the gelatine. Stir to dissolve.

2. Dilute the elderflower cordial with water or wine and add to the gelatine. Pour into 4 Champagne glasses or glass cups. Add a few berries to each and chill in the fridge for at least 4 hours or overnight until set.

Per portion: 36 kcal, 0g fat, 0g sat fat, 0g sodium, 8g carbohydrate

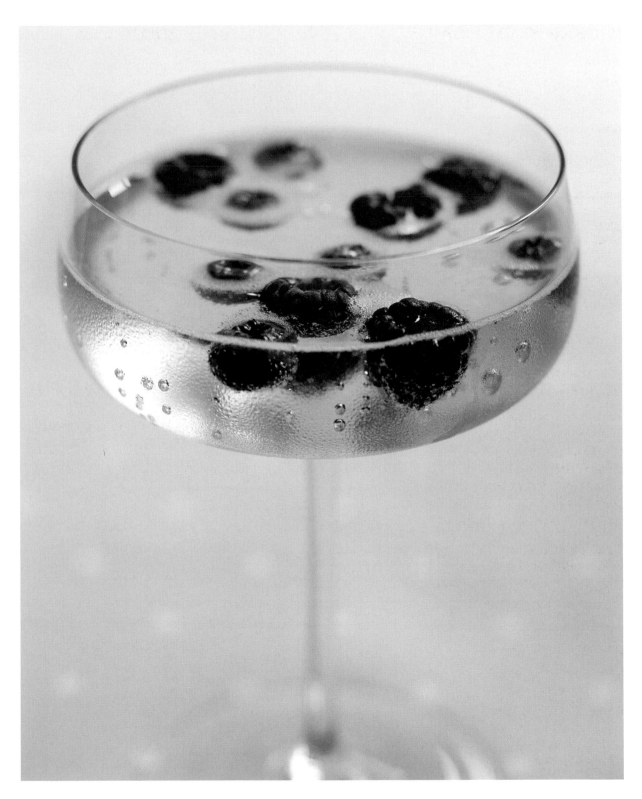

Index

A

alcohol 16, 20
almond and apricot pavlova slice 151
American sweetcorn and chilli muffins 38
apples 12, 38, 111
aubergine, red pepper, rocket and goat's cheese sandwiches 96

B

banana, raspberry and crunchy oat yogurt fool 131
barley 12, 21
beans 8, 9, 12, 13, 47, 50, 61, 79, 80
  bubble and squeak bean cakes 85
  real baked beans 51
  soya bean stew with gremolata 57
  warm mixed bean and cheese salad 97
beef 16, 100, 101
  Asian beef salad 112
  corned beef hash 111
  fruity beef casserole 101
  savoury mince with lentils 57
beetroot 10
  chunky beetroot soup with kidney beans 80
bread 8, 10, 13, 23, 38, 67
  perfect pizza dough 40
buckwheat 34
  buckwheat blinis 37
butternut squash and sausage casserole 107
butternut squash curry with coconut milk 21, 77

C

calories 14, 20, 21, 22, 26
carbohydrates 8, 9, 10, 12, 13, 15, 22, 26
carrots 10, 12
  bashed carrots with assorted seeds and lemon 83
cats' tongues 145
celeriac 19
cereals 10, 20, 22, 23
  crunchy breakfast cereal 36
cheese 8, 16, 40, 90, 96, 97, 139
  cheese and pear wraps 92
  goat's cheese, pea and dill soufflé 95
  Greek-style village salad 80

cherry and toasted pine-nut frozen yogurt 145
chicken 16, 100
  chicken livers with Moroccan spices 106
  chicken satay sticks 65
  pot-roast chicken 109
  roast garlic chicken with lemon and macadamias 108
  Thai green chicken curry 108
children 18, 19, 31, 90
chilli 38, 117
  chilli, tomato, oat and bean bake 61
chocolate, honey and sesame seed popcorn 35
chocolate semi-freddo 146
chocolate soufflés, hot 146
cholesterol 16, 18, 26
cod, prawn and sweetcorn chowder 117
corn 34, 38, 103, 117, 123
couscous 10, 21
  pumpkin couscous 43

D

dairy produce 8, 16, 90
diabetes 8, 18, 19
diets 8, 9, 14, 19
Dijon mackerel with Scandinavian potato salad 127
drinks 16
dukkah 65

E

eating out 20
eggs 8, 16, 19, 90
  pipérade 91
  poached eggs with ham, tomato and watercress 92
  scrambled eggs on grilled field mushroom 93
  Spanish tortilla 95
elderflower jellies 154
energy bars 44
entertaining 31
exercise 14

F

fat 8, 9, 16, 19, 20, 21, 26
fennel 19
figs grilled with pancetta 131
fish 8, 16, 116
  mackerel 72, 127
flour 12, 19, 21
fluids 16

food intolerances 19, 34
fruit 8, 10, 20, 22, 24–25, 101, 130
  baked breakfast fruits 133
  dried 21
  fruit salad of mango, strawberries and blueberries with fresh lime 137
  luxury fruit salad 134

G

gingerbread with pear 153
glucose 10, 14, 27
Glycaemic Index 9, 12, 13
Glycaemic Load 9, 12
  benefits 18
  calculating 13
  food tables 22–25
  health 19
  meal ideas 28–31
  reducing 20
  shopping 21
  weight loss 15, 18, 26–27
  zero-rated foods 16
grains 8, 12, 19, 34
  mixed grain jambalaya 71
Greek cherry glyko 149

H

haddock with a horseradish herb crust 120
hazelnut meringues 143
health concerns 8, 14, 18, 19
herbs 19, 21
honey 35, 37, 143
hot mochas 150
houmous 52

I

insulin 10, 12, 18, 19, 27
Iranian fruit and nut pilaff 43
irritable bowel syndrome (IBS) 8, 18, 19

K

kamut with peas, spring onions and mint 55

L

lamb 16, 100
  aromatic lamb fillet 103
  lamb chump steaks with mint mechoul 104
  lamb curry with chick peas and spinach 104
  lamb's liver with shallots and balsamic vinegar 106

leek stew 86
lemon 19, 20, 41, 83, 108
    lemon blancmanges with
        honeyed blackberries 143
lentils 8, 10, 12, 50, 57, 119
    lentil and coriander burgers 58
    spiced lentil salad with prawns
        and mint yogurt 55
liver 16, 106

M
meat 8, 16, 100
menstrual problems 19
milk 8, 10, 19, 21, 22, 90
minestrone verde 79
mint 55, 104, 123
monkfish with warm spinach salad
    124
mood 14, 18
mushrooms 19, 93

N
nutrition 8
nuts 8, 10, 15, 19, 20, 21, 64
    hazelnuts 139,143
    walnuts 67, 73, 86

O
oats 8, 10, 12, 20, 21, 34, 35
    plum oat crumble 133
    seeded oat thins 68
oils 16, 19, 64
onions 19, 55, 83
    onion, cherry tomato and curd
        cheese pizza 40

P
passion cake 153
pasta 8, 10, 12, 15, 20, 21
    one-pot pasta with potato, green
        beans and rocket 21, 79
    pasta e fagioli 51
peach and blueberry gratin 135
peaches baked with brown sugar
    and almonds 135
pears 92, 153
    pan-fried pear salad with
        hazelnuts and blue cheese 139
    pears, prunes, oranges and
        pecans in spiced port wine 134
peas 10, 12, 50, 55, 95, 104, 123
    pea guacamole 52
peppers 61, 91, 96
pineapple 10
    carpaccio of pineapple with
        spiced cherries 138

plum jam 149
plum oat crumble 133
polycystic ovary syndrome 18, 19
popcorn 21, 34, 35
pork 16, 100
    open-topped BLTs with spicy
        sweetcorn salsa 103
    pork fillet stroganoff 112
    pork, prune and apple hot pot 111
    traditional meatball stew 58
potatoes 8, 10, 20, 76, 79, 127
    baby roast potatoes 82
poultry 8, 16, 100
prawns 55, 117
    curried prawns and beans with
        cashew nuts 71
    garlic chilli prawns with papaya
        117
    prawn and leek pancakes 37
    prawn and noodle salad with
        peanut dressing 120
protein 8, 9, 15
pumpkin couscous 43

Q
quinoa 34
    fiery quinoa 44

R
raisin, rosemary and apple soda
    bread 38
rice 8, 10, 20, 21, 34
    lemon poppy seed rice 41
    Oriental Basmati rice with
        beansprouts 47
    red rice and kidney bean
        salad 47
ricotta fruit cake 154
roasted peperonata with cannellini
    beans 61

S
salt 19, 20, 21, 26, 100
scallops with crushed minted peas
    123
seabass fillets with salmoriglio and
    lentils 119
seeds 8, 12, 15, 19, 20, 21, 35, 64,
    65, 83
    seeded oat thins 68
    seeded soda bread rolls 67
shellfish 18, 116
skate with a fresh Mediterranean
    sauce 127
snack foods 25
soya 8, 19, 21, 57, 90

spices 21, 55, 103, 106, 134, 138
    spiced nut fingers 68
    spiced sponge roll with berries
        148
    spiced tabbouleh with smoked
        mackerel 72
spinach 104, 124
    Spanish-style spinach with
        walnuts and cumin 86
    spinach raita 91
stock cubes 21
storecupboard standbys 21
strawberries with vanilla ice cream
    137
strawberry porridge with oatbran,
    honey and sunflower seeds 35
sugar 8, 12, 13, 14, 15, 16, 21, 22,
    135, 142
    blood sugar 10, 18, 19, 27
    sugar and spice salmon with
        char-grilled corn salsa 123
sweet potato mash with Dijon
    mustard and spring onions 83
syndrome X 18, 19

T
tomatoes 19, 40, 61, 92
trout saltimbocca 124
tuna on warm pak choi with
    mustard seed, ginger and lime
        dressing 119
turkey 16, 100
    paprika turkey in pitta pockets
        107

V
vegetables 8, 20, 21, 22, 23–24, 76
    braised red cabbage 85
    green stew 73
    vegetable stir-fry 82

W
walnut bread 67
water 16
watermelon 10, 15
weight loss 8–9, 14, 15, 18, 26–27
wheat 19, 24

Y
yeast 19
yogurt 8, 55, 90, 131, 145
    yogurt and dill bulgur 41

Conversion table

Weight (solids)		Volume (liquids)		Length	
7g	¼oz	5ml	1 teaspoon	5mm	⅛in
10g	½oz	10ml	1 dessertspoon	1cm	½in
20g	¾oz	15ml	1 tablespoon	2cm	¾in
25g	1oz		or ½fl oz	2.5cm	1in
40g	1½oz	30ml	1fl oz	3cm	1¼in
50g	2oz	40ml	1½fl oz	4cm	1½in
60g	2 ½oz	50ml	2fl oz	5cm	2in
75g	3oz	60ml	2½fl oz	7.5cm	3in
100g	3½oz	75ml	3fl oz	10cm	4in
110g	4oz (¼lb)	100ml	3½fl oz	15cm	6in
125g	4½oz	125ml	4fl oz	18cm	7in
150g	5½oz	150ml	5fl oz (¼ pint)	20cm	8 in
175g	6oz	160ml	5½fl oz	24cm	10in
200g	7oz	175ml	6fl oz	28cm	11in
225g	8oz (½lb)	200ml	7fl oz	30cm	12in
250g	9oz	225ml	8fl oz		
275g	10oz	250ml	9fl oz		
300g	10½oz	(0.25 litre)			
310g	11oz	300ml	10fl oz (½ pint)		
325g	11½oz	325ml	11fl oz		
350g	12oz (¾lb)	350ml	12fl oz		
375g	13oz	370ml	13fl oz		
400g	14oz	400ml	14fl oz		
425g	15oz	425ml	15fl oz (¾ pint)		
450g	1lb	450ml	16fl oz		
500g (½kg)	18oz	500ml	18fl oz		
600g	1¼lb	(0.5 litre)			
700g	1½lb	550ml	19fl oz		
750g	1lb 10oz	600ml	20fl oz (1 pint)		
900g	2lb	700ml	1¼ pints		
1kg	2¼lb	850ml	1½ pints		
1.1kg	2½lb	1 litre	1¾ pints		
1.2kg	2lb 12oz	1.2 litres	2 pints		
1.3kg	3lb	1.5 litres	2 ½ pints		
1.5kg	3lb 5oz	1.8 litres	3 pints		
1.6kg	3½lb	2 litres	3½ pints		
1.8kg	4lb				
2kg	4lb 8oz				
2.25kg	5lb				
2.5kg	5lb 8oz				
3kg	6lb 8oz				

Acknowledgements

It's all too easy to pour a generous dash of olive oil into a pan before starting to fry, spread toast with lashings of butter or make a rich pudding using double cream. The GL makes you rethink all that and while creating and testing these recipes, I too was challenged with how to make food still taste good whilst following the GL rules. It isn't difficult and the result is food which seems to have a purer and fresher taste. My thanks go to Anna Helm who assisted me with great enthusiasm during all the testing and photography. It's also been a joy as ever to work with such a dedicated and capable team. (JS)

This has been a wonderful chance to address comments from both my patients and all the lovely people who read the previous book. Knowledge of GL really moves things forward and after a week of low-GL eating as I tried out recipes I lost 2kg and my husband 3kg without any difficulty. The only oil recently has been the calorie-free 'midnight variety' in writing the book. Again it has been inspirational to work with Antony, Jane and Muna. Most importantly thanks to Peter Blades for his love, help and support and also to Daisy Rose for her encouragement. (MB)

Resources

The recipes are based on ingredients purchased from supermarkets, greengrocers, small independent shops and wholefood shops. If the items you want are not in stock, try substituting another item and also try asking at the customer services desk in the supermarket to arrange to get them in for you.

For anyone with intolerances and allergies, most supermarkets produce specialist information – again ask at the customer services desk.

If you require a special diet ask a Registered Dietitian or health professional for individual advice.

Suppliers of gluten-free flours include Gluten Free Foods, Nutricia, General Dietary Ltd and Dietary Specialists. Local pharmacists may be able to help with specialist products.

Coeliac UK provides information on gluten-free diets: www.coeliac.org.uk.

Egg replacers are available from supermarkets and health food shops. Gluten Free Foods also produces an egg substitute.

Information on diabetes and diets can be obtained from Diabetes UK.

Lakeland Plastics Ltd provide a range of items for cooking and also do seeds by post: www.lakelandlimited.co.uk

Cookware that requires no fat can be obtained from Well Bake: www.wellbake.co.uk.

Further reading

Antony Worrall Thompson's GI Diet
Antony Worrall Thompson, Dr Mabel Blades and Jane Suthering
Kyle Cathie Ltd

Nutrition and Health
Dr Mabel Blades
Highfield Publications

Healthy Eating for Diabetes
Antony Worrall Thompson and Azmina Govindji
Kyle Cathie Ltd

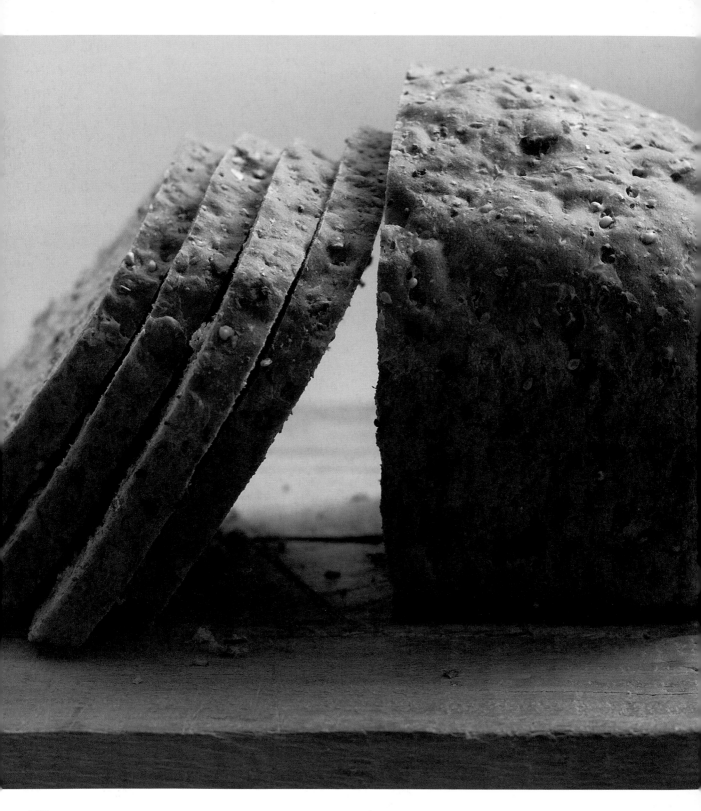